This book is to be returned on or before
the last date stamped below

MUTILATING INJURIES OF THE HAND

GROUPE D'ÉTUDE DE LA MAIN (G.E.M.)

List of Members

U.K.
D. M. Brooks (London) G. Fisk (Essex) S. H. Harrison (London) J. I. P. James (Edinburgh) F. Nicolle (London) R. G. Pulvertaft (Derby) R. H. C. Robins (Cornwall) H. G. Stack (Essex) C. B. Wynn Parry (London)

U.S.A.
A. J. Barsky (New York) R. Beasley (New York) J. Bell (Chicago) J. Boswick (Colorado) J. Boyes (California) J. Brand (California) S. Brown (California) E. Clark (California) R. Curtis (Maryland) A. E. Flatt (Iowa) J. Hunter (Philadelphia) E. Kaplan (New York) C. H. Lane (California) W. J. Littler (New York) J. W. Madden (Arizona) L. Milford (Tennessee) E. Nalebuff (Massachusetts) M. Spinner (New York) A. B. Swanson (Michigan)

Australia
M. Fahrer (Queensland) J. Hueston (Victoria) W. Morrison (Melbourne)

France
P. C. Achach (Paris) Y. Allieu (Montpellier) J-Y. Alnot (Paris) J. Aubriot (Caen) P. Banzet (Paris) J. Baudet (Bordeaux) S. Baux (Paris) J. Beres (Paris) R. Bobichon (Grenoble) J. Body (Chaumont) M. Bombart (Villeneuve St. Georges) M. Bonnel (Montpellier) J. Bonvallet (Paris) A. Borit (St. Maur les Fosses) P. Bourrel (Marseilles) J. L. Brouet (Toulon) P. de Butler (Amiens) H. Bureau (Marseilles) J. Carayon (Marseilles) A. Chancholle (Toulouse) P. Colson (Lyons) J. J. Comtet (Lyons) J. C. Dardour (Paris) P. Dautry (Paris) J. Dubousset (Clamart) J. L. Ducourtioux (Paris) C. Dufourmentel (Paris) J. Duparc (Paris) J. S. Elbaz (Paris) P. Esteve (Neuilly) G. Foucher (Strasbourg) Fourrier (Clermont-Ferrand) M. Gangolphe (Ste Foy les Lyon) R. Gay (Toulouse) A. Gilbert (Paris) J. Glicenstein (Paris) A. Goumain (Bordeaux) J. Gournet (Reims) J. Greco (Tours) C. Hamonet (Paris) S. Hauttier (Paris) F. Iselin (Paris) M. Iselin (Paris) M. Jandeaux (Vesoul) J. P. Jouglard (Aubagne) A. Julliard (Neuilly) A. Kapandji (Longjumeau) M. Kerboul (Paris) N. Kuhlmann (Beauvais) J. P. Lalardrie (Paris) F. Langlais (Paris) Lemerle (Paris) A. Lemoine (Paris) J. Lerique (Paris) C. le Quang (Paris) J. Levane (Nanterre) J. Lignon (Nantes) R. Lisfranc (Neuilly les Toul) R. Malek (Paris) M. Mansat (Toulouse) J. P. May (Paris) C. Menkes (Paris) M. Merle (Dommartin les Toul) R. Merle D'Aubigne (Acheres) J. P. Meyreuis (Toulon) J. Michon (Dommartin les Toul) C. Moitrel (Bois Guillaume) D. Morel-Fatio (Paris) R. Moully (Paris) R. Naett (Strasbourg) C. Nicoletis (Paris) J. A. Noirclerc (Collonges au Mont D'Or) P. Oger (Garches) P. Petit (Paris) M. Pierre (Carseilles) J. Pillet (Paris) J. G. Pous (Montpellier) P. Rabischong (Montpellier) J. P. Razemon (Lille) J. P. Rengeval (Paris) J. Roullet (Lyons) C. Roux (Montrouge) P. Saffar (Neuilly) T. Saucier (Grenoble) A. Sedel (Jouy en Josas) R. Souquet (Toulouse) R. Thevenin (Rouen) J. M. Thomine (Rouen) H. Tramier (Marseilles) R. Tubiana (Paris) P. Valentin (Clermont Ferrand) J. M. Vaillant (Neuilly) C. Valette (Limoges) B. Valtin (Champigny) P. Vichard (Besancon) R. Vilain (Saint Cloud)

Austria
A. Berger (Vienna) E. Trojan (Vienna) H. Millesi (Vienna)

Belgium
De Conninck (Brussels) H. Evrard (Jamioulx) H. de Frenne (Waregem) P. Van Wetter (Brussels)

Finland
K. Vainio (Heinola)

Germany
D. Buck-Gramko (Hamburg) Haimovici (Bremen) L. Mannerfelt (Villingen am Schwarzwald)

Holland
J. Bloem (Heemstede) J. F. Landsmeer (Leiden) J. Van Der Meulen (Rotterdam)

Italy
P. Bedeschi (Modena) G. Brunelli (Brescia) A. Gensini (Rome) R. Mantero (Savona) E. Morelli (Cerro Maggiore) V. Salvi (Turin)

Luxembourg
J. Y. de la Cafiniere

Spain
F. Enriquez de Salamanca (Madrid) Quintana Montero (Zaragoza)

Sweden
D. Haffajee (Lund) I. Isaksson (Linkoping) E. Moberg (Goteborg)

Switzerland
A. Chamay (Geneva) A. Graedel (Schaffhausen) U. Heim (Coire) H. Ch. Meuli (Bern) V. Meyer (Zurich) H. Nigst (Básel) C. Simonetta (Lausanne) A. O. Narakas (Lausanne) I. Poulenas (Lausanne) C. Verdan (Lausanne)

Japan
Yashimura

Algeria
Y. Martini Benkeddache (Bainen Bologhine)

Iran
Goucheh (Teheran)

Israel
M. Rousso (Jerusalem)

Libya
El Bacha

Argentina
E. Zancolli (Buenos Aires)

Venezuela
R. Contreras (Caras) E. Kamel (Caracas)

MUTILATING INJURIES OF THE HAND

Edited by D. A. Campbell Reid and the late J. Gosset

IN COLLABORATION WITH

J-Y. Alnot
P. Banzet
S. Baux
C. Dufourmentel
J. Duparc
A. Gilbert
J. Glicenstein
F. Iselin
M. Jandeaux
B. B. Joshi
R. Kanhouche
F. Langlais
C. le Quang

A. M. MacLeod
M. Mansat
P. May
J. Michon
D. Morel-Fatio
W. A. Morrison
B. McC. O'Brien
J-M. Paquin
J-P. Razemon
C. Simonetta
R. Souquet
R. Tubiana
J. Xenard

CHURCHILL LIVINGSTONE
EDINBURGH LONDON AND NEW YORK 1979

CHURCHILL LIVINGSTONE
Medical Division of Longman Group Limited

Distributed in the United States of America by Longman Inc.,
19 West 44th Street, New York, N.Y. 10036, and by associated
companies, branches and representatives throughout the world.

First edition published in French under the title *Les Mutilations
de la Main*
© Expansion Scientifique Française 1975

First edition, in English, based on the original French edition with
additional material
© Longman Group Limited 1979

ISBN 0 443 01684 4

British Library Cataloguing in Publication Data
Mutilating injuries of the hand.
— (Groupe d'Etude de la Main. Monographs; no. 3).
1. Hand—Wounds and injuries 2. Hand—Surgery
I. Reid, D A Campbell II. Gosset, J
III. Series
617'.1   RD559   78–40765

Printed in Great Britain by T. & A. Constable, Edinburgh

Contributors

J-Y. ALNOT, Hôpital Bichat, 170 Boulevard Ney, 75018 Paris

P. BANZET, 32 Rue Emile Meurier, 75016 Paris

S. BAUX, 21 Boulevard Flandrin, 75116 Paris

D. A. CAMPBELL REID, Plastic and Jaw Department, Royal Hospital Annexe, Fulwood, Sheffield S10 3TD

C. DUFOURMENTEL, 170 Rue de Courcelles, 75017 Paris

J. DUPARC, 6 Square Thiers, 75116 Paris

A. GILBERT, Hôpital Saint Vincent de Paul, 74 Avenue Denfert Rochereau, 75674 Paris

J. GLICENSTEIN, 32 Boulevard de Courcelles, 75017 Paris

J. GOSSET, 86 Rue d'Assas, 75006 Paris

F. ISELIN, 1 Rue A. Vacquerie, 75116 Paris

M. JANDEAUX, Hôpital Paul-Morel, 48 Rue Baron-Bouvier, 70014 Vesoul, Cedex

B. B. JOSHI, Department of Orthopaedic Surgery, the Mahatma Gandhi Memorial Hospital, Bombay 400 012

R. KANHOUCHE, Hôpital Jeanne d'Arc, 54200 Dommartin les Toul, Toul

F. LANGLAIS, 36 Avenue Reille, 75014 Paris

C. LE QUANG, 178 Rue de Courcelles, 75017 Paris

A. M. MacLEOD, Plastic Surgery and Microsurgery Research Units, St Vincent's Hospital, Melbourne

M. MANSAT, Hotel Dieu Saint Jacques, Service Pr Ficat, 31000 Toulouse

P. MAY, 22 Bis Rue Jouffroy, 75017 Paris

J. MICHON, Hôpital Jeanne d'Arc, 54200 Dommartin les Toul, Toul

D. MOREL-FATIO, 4 Place de Mexico, 75016 Paris

W. A. MORRISON, Plastic Surgery and Microsurgery Research Units, St Vincent's Hospital, Melbourne

B. McC. O'BRIEN, Plastic Surgery and Microsurgery Research Units, St Vincent's Hospital, Melbourne

J-M. PAQUIN, Institut de Réadaption de Nancy, Hôpital Jeanne d'Arc, 54200 Dommartin les Toul, Toul

J-P. RAZEMON, Hôpital Rabourdin, 129 Rue Royale, 59000 Lille

C. SIMONETTA, Policlinique, Chirurgical Universitaire, Avenue de la Gare, 9 Lausanne 1003, Switzerland

R. SOUQUET, 1 Bis Rue Jouxt Aygue, 31000 Toulouse

R. TUBIANA, 47 Quai des Grands Augustins, 75006 Paris

J. XENARD, Hôpital Jeanne d'Arc, 54200 Dommartin les Toul, Toul

Other titles in the G.E.M. Monograph series

Dupuytren's Disease
Edited by John T. Hueston and Raoul Tubiana
Monograph No 1 1974 Second edition 176 pages illustrated

Traumatic Nerve Lesions of the Upper Limb
Edited by J. Michon and Erik Moberg
Monograph No 2 1974 124 pages illustrated

Series editor: R. Tubiana

Contents

INTRODUCTION

D. A. Campbell Reid

The mutilated hand presents a challenge to all surgeons concerned in the management of hand injuries. The primary care of such injuries ideally should be by experienced hand surgeons. This, however, is by no means always the case but should be the eventual goal towards which we are slowly moving. In this country, the primary management of hand trauma is undertaken very largely either by the orthopaedic surgeon or the plastic surgeon. Within both these specialties, surgeons are being increasingly trained in hand surgery and participate in the overall accident and emergency services which cover the whole country. This is good but there is still a long way to go. All too often, fresh hand injuries are dealt with primarily by young, inexperienced surgeons. They will almost certainly know the basic principles from what they have read, but the putting into practice of such knowledge, when confronted with a mutilating injury to the hand, is quite another matter. Even to those experienced in dealing with primary hand trauma, these are the most difficult and challenging injuries. Furthermore, the whole future of the hand so injured may well depend upon the expertise with which the primary care is undertaken. The majority of these cases will require later reconstructive measures and these will be rendered more effective if the primary aim of clean healing has kept scar tissue to a minimum.

The primary management of the skin defect is undoubtedly the most important aspect of these cases. The surgeon performing the primary repair, therefore, should be sufficiently versed in this aspect of hand surgery to be in a position to tackle such a case with confidence. There is no doubt that some practical training in the techniques of skin replacement is a most valuable asset to the hand surgeon. Rotating registrar appointments are now widespread and provide a means for the trainee surgeon to spend a period of say six months in a plastic surgery unit. Close co-operation between the orthopaedic and plastic surgical specialties is another feature to-day which is contributing towards more efficient care in these injuries.

This book deals with the primary care and secondary reconstruction of mutilating injuries of the hand. In primary management particular emphasis is laid on the importance of providing skin with normal sensibility on important tactile surfaces.

Replantation of amputated digits has now become a practical reality with the development of microvascular techniques. Our aim should be the provision of facilities for replantation in a hand surgery service. Whether, initially, this should be in just a few centres or in every major centre is debatable. With the increasing use of microvascular techniques for free flap transfers in various centres it would seem appropriate to have a team available for emergency replantation in such a centre.

Secondary reconstruction in the mutilated hand also has much to offer and many of the following chapters are devoted to this aspect. Contributions by French hand surgeons form the bulk of them and many of these were originally presented during a symposium held by the Groupe d'Etude de la Main. Some of these have been modified and brought up to date whilst other contributions have been added. It is hoped that the combined experience of the various contributors to this work on the difficult subject of the mutilated hand will prove of value to those called upon to treat these challenging cases.

ACKNOWLEDGEMENTS

Many of the chapters in this book are based on papers originally written in French. The work of translation proved formidable and I am most indebted to my wife, Joyce, for undertaking the major part of this task. Others who helped in this aspect were Dr J. L. Rushton, M.A., Ph.D., of Sheffield, Dr Romain Vanwyck of Liège and my daughter, Annette (now Mrs J. E. C. Peters). My grateful thanks are accorded to them all.

Certain illustrations are reproduced by courtesy of the following: the Editor of the *British Journal of Plastic Surgery* (Figs. 1.1, 1.2, 1.7 and 15.10); the Editor of the *Journal of Bone and Joint Surgery* (Fig. 15.4) and Butterworths (London), Publishers (Figs. 15.3 and 15.7).

My wife also helped me enormously with proof reading and preparation of the index. I wish to thank her for this and for having had to accept long periods when I was immured during the preparation of this book.

Finally, I wish to thank Miss Zelda Gladwin, Mrs Eileen Woodthorpe, Mrs Jeanette Marriott and Mrs Mary Walker, all of whom have participated in typing the manuscript. I am most grateful to them all.

Regrettably, Professor Gosset's death was announced just before this book went to press.

1. THE SEVERELY MUTILATED HAND

D. A. Campbell Reid

CLASSIFICATION

Mutilating injuries of the hand may be arbitrarily grouped according to the part of the hand predominantly involved. Thus the following groups may be detailed:

I. DORSAL INJURIES

These involve the skin, extensor tendons and the metacarpals and/or phalanges, with or without amputation of digits. The overall outlook is relatively favourable since the important tactile surface of the hand is spared.

II. PALMAR INJURIES

There is involvement of skin, flexor tendons, digital nerves and bones, with or without amputation of digits. These injuries present a much more difficult challenge because of loss of tactile surfaces and owing to the more complex problem of restoring function to flexor tendons.

III. RADIAL HEMIAMPUTATION

These are particularly serious injuries because of the loss of thumb and therefore of the vital opposition mechanism.

IV. ULNAR HEMIAMPUTATION

These injuries are not so serious from a functional point of view as the individual will retain a grasping mechanism.

V. DISTAL AMPUTATION

This results in the so-called phalangeal or metacarpal hand. The possibility of reconstructing a functioning pinch depends on the level of loss. The more proximal the injury, the less likely is one to achieve an acceptable result.

PRIMARY MANAGEMENT OF THE SEVERELY MUTILATED HAND

INITIAL EVALUATION

It is important to undertake a critical evaluation of the hand when the patient is first seen. At the time of injury it may be obvious that the hand is beyond salvage and primary amputation will be required. The level at which this is undertaken will depend on local skin available. There is a tendency towards conservatism nowadays and provided one can cover the stump with a good palmar flap one may amputate through the carpus. If this is not possible, the hand may be disarticulated at the wrist or amputated through the lower forearm.

There will, however, be borderline cases where initial conservatism with a view to reconstruction of a grasping organ, should be practised. Experience has shown that such an approach has, on occasion, proved to have been entirely justified (Reid, 1972). If it fails, nothing will have been lost, provided efforts to achieve a functional result are not prolonged.

Another factor which is not easy to assess at the time of injury is the psychological one. A sudden mutilating injury to the hand apart from its severe physical effect must also have a considerable psychological effect on the patient. One should explain fully to him what one hopes to achieve by treatment, and thus encourage him at a time when he may be apprehensive and depressed about his future prospects.

Should the patient present with bilateral mutilation, every effort must be directed to providing some degree of usefulness to one hand. A reconstructed hand, provided it can grasp and has some sensibility, is better than an artificial one.

AIM OF TREATMENT

The basic aim of treatment in a severely mutilated hand is to provide the hand with a functioning pincer for the provision of grasping. The ideal aim is to achieve prehension, which is a more complex mechanism combining a functioning pinch with sensibility. The steps taken to achieve this will be discussed in detail and illustrated by reference to cases falling into the various classified groups already mentioned.

The main requirements for successful reconstruction are:

1. *Good skin cover*. Primary skin cover is a basic necessity in mutilating injuries to exclude infection and ensure healing with minimal scarring. This is not only important for the early result but may be essential to the success of later reconstructive procedures e.g., tendon grafting or transfer, nerve repair or grafting, bone grafting etc.

2. *Provision of motion and creation of the functioning pinch*. Initially this may depend on the stabilisation of parts and the correct placing of elements of the pinch. Later it may be necessary to undertake tendon transfers or grafts or to lengthen parts by bone grafts or pollicisation.

3. *Provision of skin with good sensibility*. The aim should be for the important tactile areas to be covered with skin of good sensibility and gnostic function as described by Moberg (1960). This may be achieved by rearrangement of local skin, use of filleted finger flaps or later by transfer of neurovascular island flaps from elsewhere in the hand or by pollicisation.

CAUSATION OF INJURY

Mutilating injuries may be caused in the following ways:

1. *Explosive injuries*. Grenade injuries in wartime; deto-

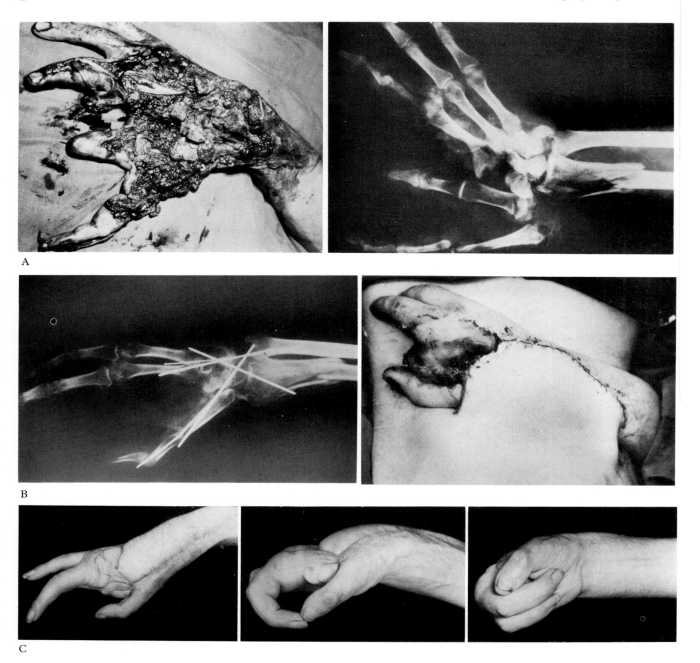

Figure 1.1
A, Severe Group I injury.
B, Kirschner wire fixation. Filleted finger flap and abdominal flap for cover.
C, Functional result.

nators and home-made 'bombs' in peace-time. The sodium chlorate 'bombs' described by McGregor and Jackson (1969) come into this category. The letter-bombs, all too familiar as a terrorist weapon, are another source of such injuries. Bilateral mutilations may occur in these explosive injuries.

2. *Lacerating injuries.* These are usually caused by electrically-driven circular saws or power-driven coal cutting machines.

3. *Crushing injuries.* Industrial presses.

4. *Burns.* Particularly electric burns. High tension current causes the most extensive injuries which may be bilateral.

DETAILED MANAGEMENT OF INDIVIDUAL CASES

It is important to remember that the final outcome of a severely mutilated hand may well depend upon the initial management. It is in the primary treatment that skin cover is all important. The aim of primary skin cover whether by direct suture, free skin graft or skin flap depending on the indication in each case, is to ensure clean healing.

Where there is skeletal disruption, the first essential in repair is to achieve stability of the bony framework upon which the soft tissue reconstruction may be built.

GROUP I INJURIES

A typical case is shown (Fig. 1.1A) where a man aged 30 caught his right hand in multiple grinding wheels. Kirschner wires were used to achieve skeletal stability. First of all, the thumb was fixed in an abducted and opposed position and the flail 4th and 5th metacarpals which were dislocated ulnarwards, were stabilised by similar wires. Once having achieved bony stability one has a firm basis on which to build up the soft tissue repair. The type of skin replacement will depend on the local condition in each case, nature of the bed, exposed structures, etc. In this particular case, the patient's index finger was not viable and had to be removed whereas the middle finger, which was completely disorganised skeletally but fully viable, was filleted to provide useful cover to the web between thumb and ring finger and to cover the exposed extensor tendons to ring and little fingers. A further advantage of such a flap is that it provides good sensibility to an important area. The remaining defect was resurfaced by a direct abdominal flap (Fig. 1.1B). The only subsequent reconstruction necessary in this case was to restore wrist extension by tendon grafts. The extensor indicis and extensor digitorum tendons to index finger in the forearm were used as motor tendons. They were extended by plantaris grafts which were attached distally to the dorsum of the hand. This procedure allowed the patient to extend his wrist to the neutral position. This combined with a satisfactory gripping function (Fig. 1.1C) enabled him to return to full employment after 8 months. He has been fully employed for the past 7 years.

The psychological trauma suffered by this young man was enormous. Once he became aware, however, that he had a functioning hand again, his outlook changed dramatically. He was completely rehabilitated, cheerful and anxious to get back to work. He was able to resume all his normal activities.

Another case in the same group concerned a man of 55 who sustained a severe crush injury to his right hand when it was trapped beneath his car which overturned in an accident. It was necessary to summon the fire brigade in order to lift the car and release the trapped hand. On admission he presented as shown (Fig. 1.2A). Again in this case, skeletal stability was achieved by Kirschner wires (Fig. 1.2B). The middle finger, though sustaining much loss of bone, had intact flexor and extensor tendons. The ring finger was filleted to provide major skin cover for the back of the hand. Later a bone graft from the iliac crest was used to reconstruct the greater part of the 3rd metacarpal (Fig. 1.2C). One was able to operate through the filleted finger flap and no additional skin cover was required. The bone graft became well incorporated and a good pinch and power grip were restored (Fig. 1.2D). This case illustrates the value of initial conservatism which led to the saving of a most useful finger. As is well known in crush injuries, tendons frequently survive intact.

An interesting psychological change was also observed in this patient. At the time, he held an important executive position and during the period in which he was unable to use his hand for normal activities he appeared indifferent to his business which suffered as a result. Once he was again able to use his hand for writing, driving etc., he soon regained his vigour and initiative.

GROUP II INJURIES

These are treated on similar lines. Skin cover is achieved by free skin grafts whenever possible but if the circumstances are unsuitable a flap will have to be used. The main principle is to achieve primary healing. Should this be by means of a free graft it may well be necessary later to replace this by a flap to open out the palm or prior to undertaking tendon reconstruction. A case is shown (Fig. 1.3) where a tubed pedicle was used for this purpose. A good alternative method of skin cover is by use of a groin flap described by McGregor and Jackson (1972). This may be used as a primary measure and has advantages over a direct abdominal flap in that it gives more freedom for movement of the hand on account of its longer pedicle and positioning of the hand is easier and more comfortable for the patient.

GROUP III INJURIES

Sometimes it is possible by relatively simple procedures to produce a definitive result at the time of primary treatment (London, 1961). A man aged 48 had his left hand crushed by a forge hammer (Fig. 1.4A). Thumb, index and middle fingers were amputated. It was possible to cover most of the thumb stump with local skin. In addition to bone involvement of the index metacarpal there was also a considerable skin defect. The skin defect also exposed the 3rd metacarpal. The potential of these metacarpals for a possible future pollicisation was therefore vitiated and they were amputated proximally. Free skin grafting was used to cover a residual defect in the thumb web, extending on to the tactile surface of the thumb. Subsequently, this area on the thumb was replaced by rotating a

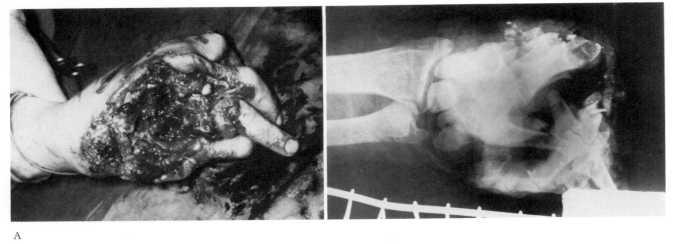

A

B   C

Figure 1.2
A, Another Group I injury with gross damage to metacarpals.
B, Skeletal stability. Note deficiency of 3rd metacarpal. The 4th ray has been removed.
C, Bone graft to 3rd metacarpal.
D, Functional result demonstrated.

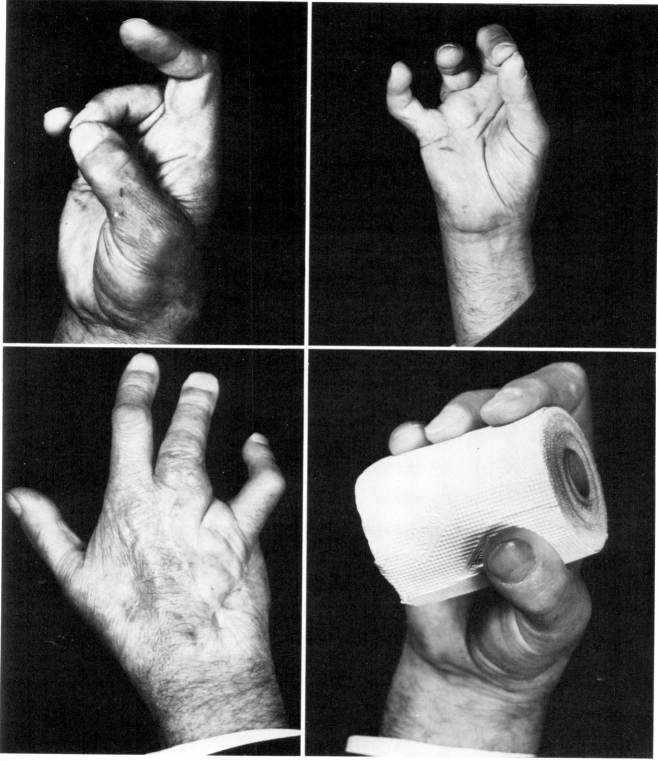

D

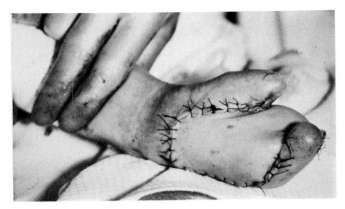

Figure 1.3
Group II injury after secondary flap replacement.

flap with radial nerve innervation giving a good functional result (Fig. 1.4B). The shortness of the thumb is overcome to a certain extent by the depth of the cleft between it and the remaining two finger elements.

GROUP IV INJURIES

The patient whose hand is illustrated (Fig. 1.5A) is a general surgeon who had sustained ulnar hemiamputation when his right hand was run over by a train with loss of the 4th and 5th digital rays. Primary management necessitated skin cover by means of a direct abdominal flap. The only secondary procedure was a multiple Z-plasty on the adjoining scar between the flap and the palm of the hand. He has been able to resume his career using specially made rubber gloves (Fig. 1.5B). The case illustrates the good function which may be obtained in such an injury.

GROUP V INJURIES

A schoolboy aged 15 sustained very severe injuries to both hands when a home-made bomb exploded prematurely. The right hand was virtually blown off and there was nothing useful which could be saved. Primary amputation through the forearm was undertaken. The condition of the left hand was as shown (Fig. 1.6A). The thumb, although partially degloved, was skeletally intact. All four fingers were lost with the exception of part of the proximal phalanx of the little finger. The metacarpals of index, middle and ring fingers were exposed in the wound. Primary skin cover was achieved by a large direct abdominal flap, the secondary defect being resurfaced with a split skin graft (Fig. 1.6B). The flap was divided 3 weeks later and healed uneventfully. After a period of 4 months, phalangisation was undertaken giving an excellent range of thumb movement (Fig. 1.6C). There was also good movement in the remains of the little finger enabling him to grasp even small objects between it and the thumb. He had a prosthesis fitted to his right forearm and this, combined with his reconstructed left hand, enabled him to undertake virtually any function (Fig. 1.6D). By sheer determination this young man set about

overcoming his enormous disability right from the start. He learned to drive a car and went to university where he obtained his degree. He became a skilled draughtsman and gained a major national award for his part in designing one of the new Colleges of Technology.

This case illustrates the importance of reconstructing at least one hand in a severe bilateral mutilating injury. It also reiterates the importance of primary skin cover. In this instance a flap was mandatory to save as much as possible of the hand. This ensured the restoration of a functioning pinch.

DEFINITIVE RECONSTRUCTION OF THE SEVERELY MUTILATED HAND

Severe mutilating injuries frequently involve the thumb and some form of thumb reconstruction will usually be required. As the thumb loss may be associated with partial loss of other digits, the use of one of these in reconstruction has made pollicisation a valuable procedure. The author, in describing his experience of pollicisation (Reid, 1969) noted that in the 13 traumatic cases there were associated mutilations of other digits in nine cases and pollicisation was undertaken using the index finger in six cases, the middle in two and the ring finger in one. This experience has since been extended and is presented with other contributions on pollicisation in subsequent chapters.

The use of the neurovascular island flap in mutilating injuries has been described by several authors, Reid (1960, 1966), Pulvertaft (1966), Tubiana *et al.* (1966) and Tubiana (1970). To demonstrate the value of this procedure a typical case is shown. This was a boy of 15 who presented for reconstruction of his right hand following a severe mutilating injury by a circular saw 8 months previously (Fig. 1.7A). Reconstruction was undertaken by lengthening the thumb using a reversed Gillies 'cocked hat' procedure as suggested by Barron (1963). The 2nd metacarpal was used to lengthen the thumb but instead of covering the secondary defect on the thumb with a free skin graft, a neurovascular island flap taken from the ulnar aspect of the little finger stump was mobilised and brought through to provide sensation, on the tactile surface of the thumb. Further phalangisation was later undertaken together with a rotation/angulation osteotomy of the 5th metacarpal. This provided a pincer action as shown (Fig. 1.7B).

SUMMARY

Severe mutilations of the hand seen at the time of initial trauma usually present complex problems of repair involving all the structures of the hand. Provision of skin cover and bony stability are the first priorities. Initial conservatism should be practised in cases where the survival of an important structure is in doubt. In cases of bilateral mutilation, every effort should be made to preserve function in one hand. The quality of sensibility on tactile surfaces is stressed.

In later reconstruction of the severely mutilated hand, the value of pollicising a mutilated digit has been mentioned.

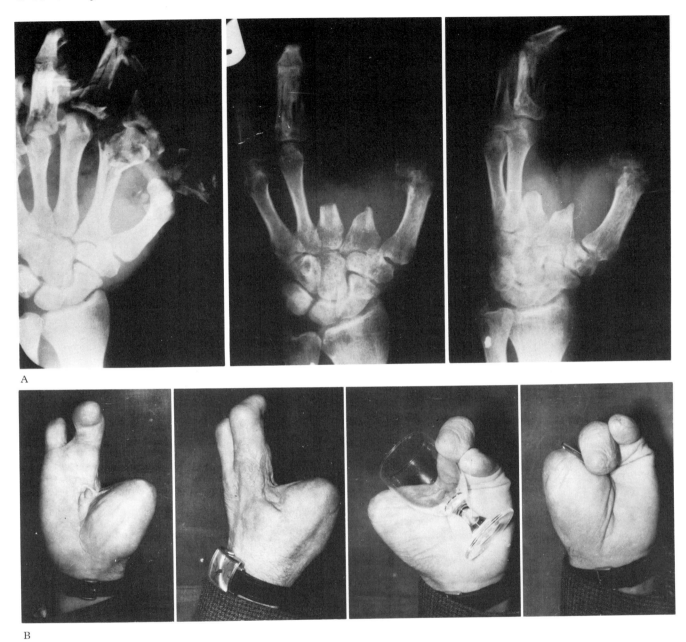

A

B

Figure 1.4
A, X-ray of a Group III injury before and after primary surgery.
B, Result of conservative surgery.

B

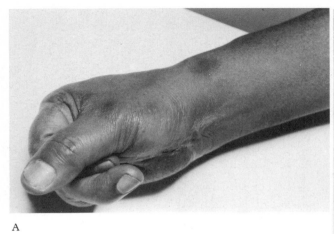

A

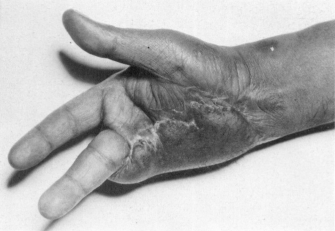

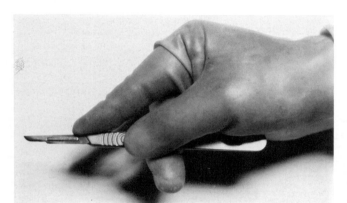

B

Figure 1.5
A, Result of treatment of a Group IV injury by means of a primary abdominal flap.
B, Patient (a general surgeon) wearing specially made rubber glove.

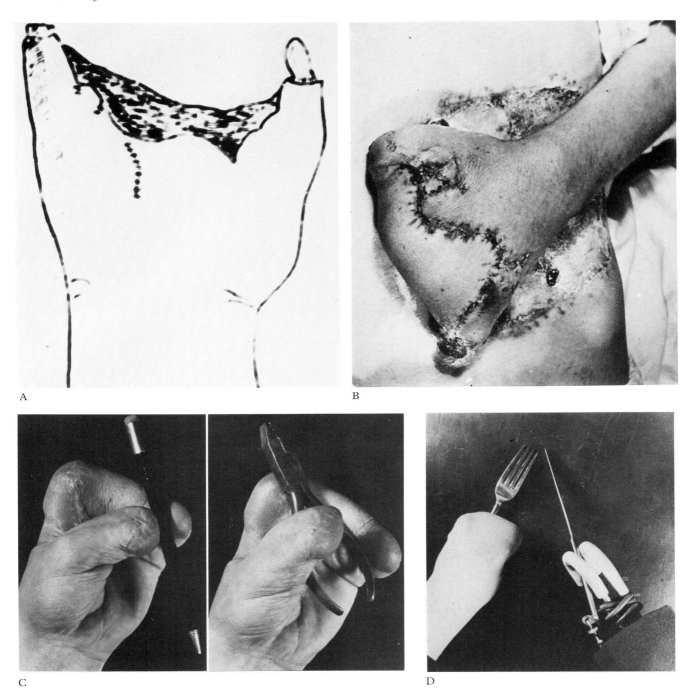

Figure 1.6
A, A Group V injury following an explosion.
B, Primary abdominal flap to cover defect.
C, Result of phalangisation.
D, Prosthesis fitted to right forearm.

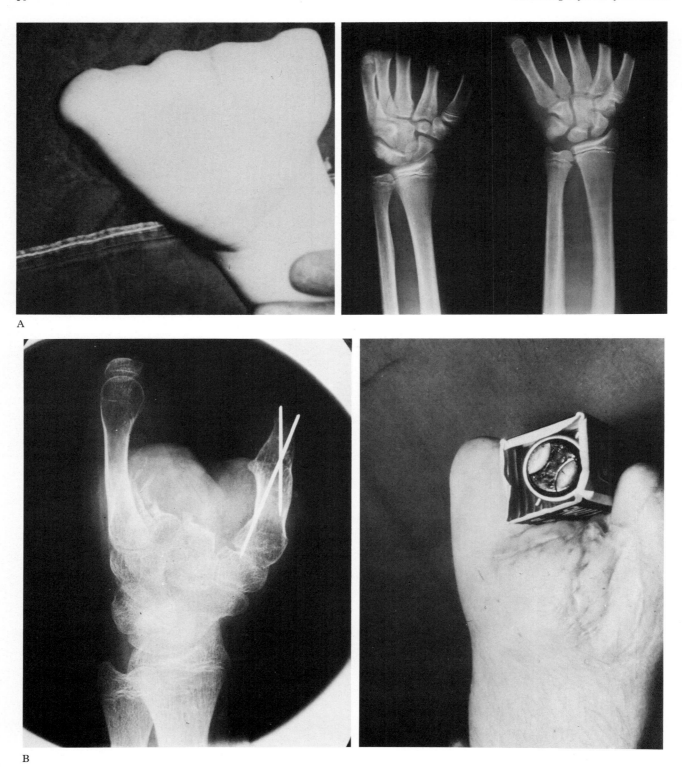

Figure 1.7
A, Metacarpal hand prior to reconstruction.
B, Result of reconstruction, providing crude grasp.

Another means of providing skin with gnostic sensation viz., by transference of a neurovascular island flap, has also been employed.

Important psychological changes have been observed in patients with severe hand mutilations and the way these have responded to effective surgical reconstruction has been gratifying.

BIBLIOGRAPHY

BARRON, J. N. (1963). Personal communication.

LONDON, P. S. (1961). Simplicity of approach to treatment of the injured hand. *Journal of Bone and Joint Surgery*, **43B,** 454.

McGREGOR, I. A. & JACKSON, I. T. (1969). Sodium chlorate bomb injuries of the hand. *British Journal of Plastic Surgery*, **22,** 16.

McGREGOR, I. A. & JACKSON, I. T. (1972). The groin flap. *British Journal of Plastic Surgery*, **25,** 3.

MOBERG, E. (1960). Evaluation of sensibility in the hand. *Surgical Clinics of North America*, **40,** 357.

PULVERTAFT, R. G. (1966). *Congress Soc. Int. Chir. Orthop Traumat* p. 189.

REID, D. A. CAMPBELL (1960). Reconstruction of the thumb. *Journal of Bone and Joint Surgery*, **42B,** 648.

REID, D. A. CAMPBELL (1966). Clinical surgery. *The Hand* p. 144. London: Butterworth.

REID, D. A. CAMPBELL (1969). Pollicisation—an appraisal. *The Hand*, **1,** 27.

REID, D. A. CAMPBELL (1972). An unusual mutilating injury of the hand. *British Journal of Plastic Surgery*, **25,** 53.

TUBIANA, R., STACK, H. G. & HAKSTIAN, R. W. (1966). Restoration of prehension after severe mutilations of the hand. *Journal of Bone and Joint Surgery*, **48B,** 455.

TUBIANA, R. (1970). Reconstruction after traumatic mutilations of the hand. *Injury*, **2,** 127.

2. SENSORY FLAPS FOR THE DEGLOVED MUTILATED HAND

B. B. Joshi

Mutilated hands in industrial workers are often the result of their being caught in the mobile parts of machines. These accidents not only cause damage to the skin and soft tissues but also make a pulp of the digits necessitating amputation and leaving behind a mutilated hand with varied dismembered degloved parts. These include degloved remnants of the fingers and thumb which must be saved to preserve the basic function of a hand capable of pinch and grasp. The degloved remnants require replacement of skin by free grafts or flaps. Such skin cover over the volar distal surface and stumps gives poor sensory quality and also suffers from trophic disturbances due to impaired blood supply. Since the hand is not only an organ of grasp but also of touch, the mutilating injury of a hand with degloved elements forms a special challenge to the surgeon in providing innervated skin for strategic areas of grasp and pinch. A salvaged prehensile hand unit should be able to stand comparison with the artificial limb. In severe degloving injuries there may not be sufficient innervated skin for restoration of full sensation but endeavour should be made to restore as much as can be accomplished by re-alignment of the available skin.

The hand has a definite pattern of distribution of the nerves with well demarcated areas of supply by various branches of the main nerves. It is also a known fact that anomalous nerve supply is not an uncommon feature and there is a great amount of overlapping of the nerves. Before considering the transfer of innervated skin, it is essential to chart the sensory pattern in the remaining degloved hand by means of nerve blocks. These are tested individually and in combination to demarcate the zone of their supply and the areas of overlapping. This will help to plan the operations rationally.

From the anatomical study of the nerve supply of the hand and digits four distinct areas of transferable skin emerge for utilisation in sensory rehabilitation of the degloved hand:
1. Remains of the palmar digital skin distal to the palmar digital creases based on individual palmar digital nerves.
2. Radial innervated dorsal skin over the 2nd metacarpal and base of the proximal phalanx of the index finger.
3. Innervated dorsal skin of the fingers.
4. Median or ulnar innervated segments of palmar skin.

1. REMAINS OF THE PALMAR DIGITAL SKIN DISTAL TO THE PALMAR DIGITAL CREASES BASED ON INDIVIDUAL PALMAR DIGITAL NERVES (FIG. 2.1)

Since they usually have one or more digital vessels and nerves still intact in them, these digital skin remains can be utilised in various ways for re-alignment of the sensory skin at important areas of the fingers where they can be more effective in perception:

(a) The proximally based sliding flap (Moberg, 1964) can be a very useful procedure. By keeping the metacarpo-phalangeal joint flexed even the palmar skin flap can be advanced appreciably. The resultant flexion contracture is relieved at a second stage by a transverse incision, converting the distal part to a neurovascular island of sensory skin.

Further advance of this flap can be achieved by loosening the neurovascular bundles proximally. The resultant gap in the skin is resurfaced by free skin graft or by adjustment of any locally available skin. Figure 2.2 shows an example of a problematic case. The degloved index finger remnant was conserved by a primary tubed flap (Fig. 2.2A). Sensation was provided by sliding the palmar skin from the thenar region on to the index finger stump held in a flexed position (Fig. 2.2B) and later correcting the flexion deformity. Additional migration of the innervated skin was achieved utilising neurovascular pedicles (Fig. 2.2C and D).

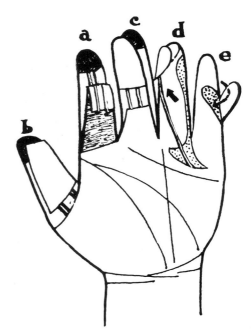

Figure 2.1
Line drawing of the various sensory flaps for degloved finger segments or stumps. *Key :* (a) proximally based palmar sliding flap; (b) rotation and advancement of palmar flap on neurovascular attachment; (c) island flap based on both neurovascular bundles; (d) island flap based on single neurovascular pedicle; (e) dorsolateral rotation flap.

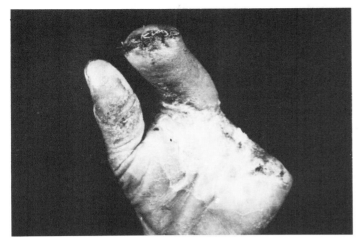

A

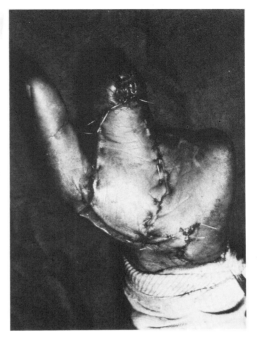

B

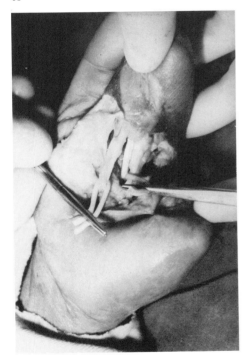

C

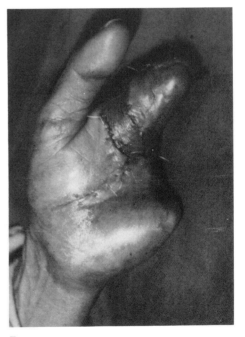

D

Figure 2.2
A, Degloved remains of index finger covered by tubed pedicle flap.
B, Advancement of thenar palmar skin by sliding over the stump. The umbrella fashion of neurovascular attachment ensures its survival as an island flap.
C, Method of conversion of the distal part of this flap into a creeping island flap with neurovascular attachment.
D, Final result.

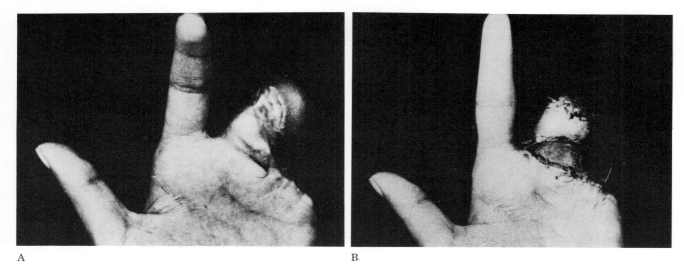

A   B.

Figure 2.3
A, Middle finger stump salvaged by pedicle flap skin.
B, Advancement of the remains of the sensory skin on neurovascular pedicle with coverage of the donor area by locally available skin.

(b) Remains of the volar digital skin may also be utilised as a rotation flap to bring innervated skin over the distal parts of the stumps (Fig. 2.1B). Such a flap may be raised on a single neurovascular bundle. The proximal donor site is covered by a free graft or by transfer of the nearby available skin from the dorsum of the same finger (Fig. 2.3A and B). An alternative is to use a second rotation flap from the radially innervated dorsal skin over the 2nd metacarpal region as in the case of the thumb (Joshi, 1970) or a single stage proximally based cross finger flap from the dorsum of the adjacent finger.

(c) The remains of the volar digital skin may also be migrated distally as an island flap utilising both neurovascular bundles (O'Brien, 1966) (Fig. 2.1C) or as a dorsolateral island flap on a single volar neurovascular pedicle (Fig. 2.1D) to advance and rotate it in a volar direction (Joshi, 1974) to cover the strategic area over the stumps of the fingers.

(d) These volar digital remains may also be utilised as an island flap to a different finger (Littler, 1959; Tubiana and Duparc, 1961). The sensory skin can be redistributed to the remaining fingers from any available volar digital skin. This could also be utilised to transfer sensibility over the reconstructed parts of the mutilated hand by osteoplastic techniques.

2. RADIAL INNERVATED DORSAL SKIN OVER THE 2ND METACARPAL AND BASE OF THE PROXIMAL PHALANX OF THE INDEX FINGER (FIG. 2.4A AND B)

This skin has neurovascular bundles of the dorsal digital branches of the radial nerve and vessels. It is amenable for transfer to provide sensation over the palmar aspect of the thumb (Holevich, 1963) or to the base of the index finger (Boyes, 1964). Such a transfer could also be useful in providing sensation on the index finger stump or in the 1st web space for adduction pinch of the thumb. Its utilisation as an inner-

vated cross finger flap for the thumb with transposition of the neurovascular bundle at the time of detachment makes it a more reliable procedure (Wilson, 1964; Adamson *et al.*, 1967; Brailler and Horton, 1969; Gaul, 1969).

3. DORSAL INNERVATED SKIN OVER THE OTHER FINGERS

This skin has a limited use. The dorsal skin may be transposed anteriorly as a proximally based flap on the finger or thumb, especially over the middle and proximal segments in massive avulsion injuries of the palm of the hand and fingers (Fig. 2.5).

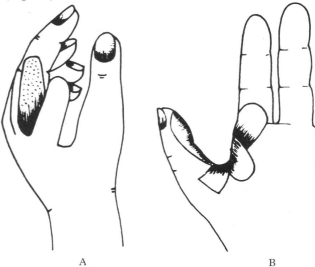

A   B

Figure 2.4
A, Line drawings of radial innervated dorsal flap from 2nd metacarpal and proximal part index finger.
B, The sites where this flap could be gainfully utilised.

The cutaneous nerves to the dorsum of the fingers have a segmental distribution. The segment over the proximal phalanx is supplied by the terminal branches of the dorsal nerves of the hand, i.e. by radial nerve and dorsal branch of the ulnar nerve. The dorsal skin over the proximal phalanges can also be used as a single stage, proximally based, cross finger flap with intact nerve supply over the volar aspect of the proximal phalanges of the adjacent finger or at the web of the fingers. The flap may also be used in combination with advancement of available volar distal skin and would thus provide the donor site with sensitive skin (Fig. 2.6A).

The skin over the two distal segments is supplied by dorsal branches of the volar digital nerves of the fingers. On the radial aspect of the index and middle fingers and on the ulnar aspect of the little finger a specific dorsal branch is given off at the level of the base of the proximal phalanx to supply the middle segment of these fingers (Milford, 1964). We can apply this anatomical fact to convert the radially based standard cross finger flaps from the dorsum of the middle segment of the middle finger to the volar aspect of the index finger into a sensory flap by transposing this dorsal branch of the volar digital nerve along with the flap (Fig. 2.7). As the nerve supply of such a flap is kept intact, this procedure could be utilised to supply innervated skin over the index finger in circumstances where the volar skin available for transfer is in short supply due to amputation of ulnar digits.

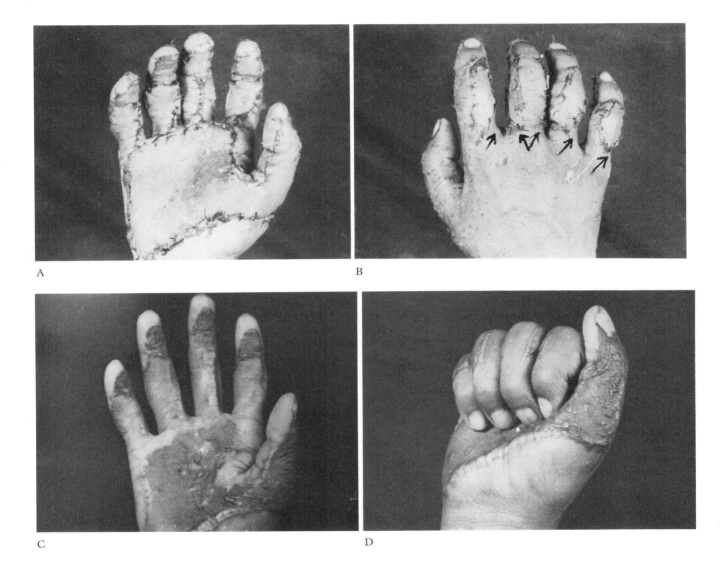

A B

C D

Figure 2.5
A and B, Dorsal rotation flaps from various fingers used in degloving injury of the hand over the proximal and middle segments of the fingers. C and D, Final result.

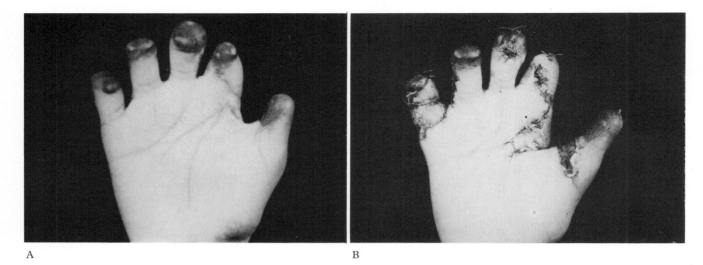

A   B

Figure 2.6
A, Degloved stump of a mutilated hand.
B, Illustrates the utilisation of the local dorsal skin for providing the sensory skin over the donor site of the advancement flaps.
   In the case of index finger stump, this was achieved by a dorsal flap of the proximal phalanx. The little finger stump had a single staged, proximally based, cross finger flap from the dorso-ulnar aspect of the ring finger stump at the donor site of the advanced local neurovascular island flap.

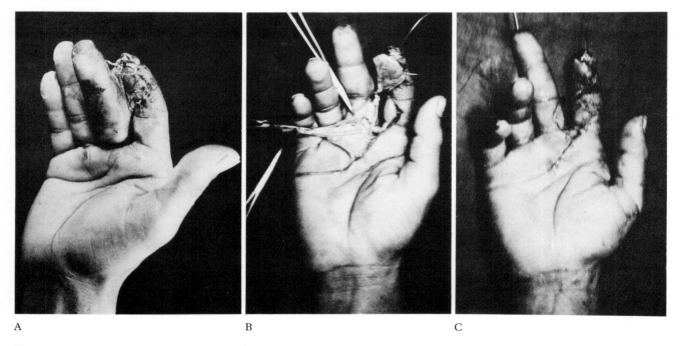

A   B   C

Figure 2.7
A, Cross finger flap from the middle segment of the middle finger over the pulp of the index finger.
B, Dissection to isolate its nerve supply i.e., dorsal branch of the volar digital nerve to the radial side.
C, Completion of the operation.

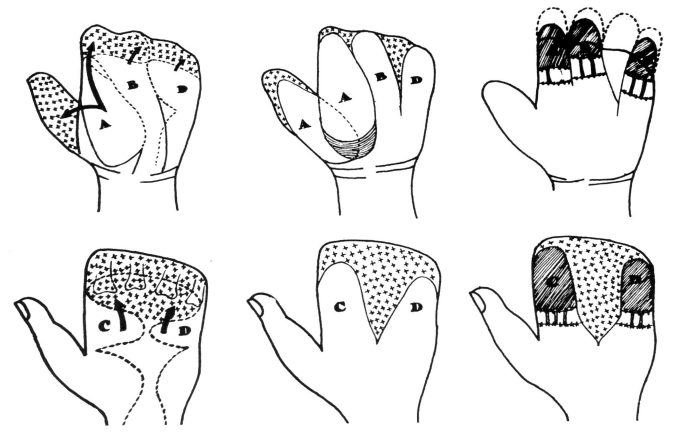

Figure 2.8
Line drawing of various flaps utilised for advancement by rotation, sliding and probable conversion into island flaps distally as staged operations. *Key:* (A) thenar flap and palmar flap; (B) ulnar based median innervated flap; (C) radial based median innervated flap; (D) ulnar innervated flap.

4. MEDIAN AND ULNAR INNERVATED SEGMENTS OF THE PALM (FIG. 2.8)

The area supplied by median and ulnar nerves is well known and conforms to a well defined pattern though some variations are not uncommon. The use of a rotation flap to advance skin from the palm was suggested by Nicolle *et al.* (1966). They did not include the common palmar digital nerves in their flaps but relied entirely on sensory overlap from a diffuse plexus in the palm formed by cutaneous branches of the terminal part of the radial nerve, the lateral cutaneous nerve of the forearm, the medial cutaneous nerve of the forearm and the palmar cutaneous branch of the median nerve. It is felt that retention of the common volar digital vessels and nerves in such flaps makes them both safer and more reliable in the quality of sensation. The flaps described here are essentially neurovascular, based on specific common digital vessels and nerves, and can be converted into islands of innervated skin on neurovascular pedicles. The manner of their advancement is based on the 'safety first' principle. The initial advancement is gained by the rotation of the flaps along with the nerves and vessels of the flaps ensheathed in them and

by flexing the finger joints. The degloved remnants having previously been covered with skin flaps one may then plan shifting the innervated flaps. After healing has been obtained and the tissues have adjusted, the distal part of these segments is converted into islands of sensory skin by releasing the flexion contracture and loosening the neurovascular pedicle proximally, so as to permit further advancement and adjustment at the strategic areas. We have named this method of obtaining advancement as 'creeping advancement' because the flaps are not allowed to lose the support of the surrounding attachments.

The palmar skin can be utilised in four different ways:

(a) *Thenar region and base of the index finger*. This segment (Fig. 2.9A) is based on the palmar branches of the median nerve and other cutaneous twigs from digital branches to the index finger. Apart from the palmar cutaneous branch of the median nerve which enters the flap proximally as a distinct branch, the other branches from the median nerve enter it centrally. The flap is outlined by extension of the thenar crease line to the base of the index finger so as to include one or two common palmar digital branches of the median nerve.

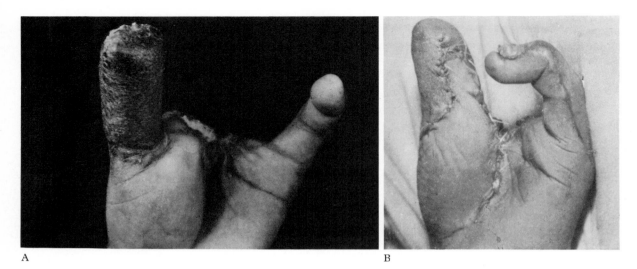

A   B

Figure 2.9
A and B, Illustrate the utilisation of thenar flap over the reconstructed thumb.

This flap is utilised mainly to provide sensation over the palmar aspect of the thumb. When the index finger has been amputated as is shown in Figure 2.9 the flap may be used to introduce sensation to a thumb reconstructed by tubed pedicle. In this case the sole remaining finger was a damaged little finger. This flap may also be utilised as a sliding flap since the main nerve and vessels enter it like an umbrella. The cutaneous branch of the median nerve entering it proximally can be identified and mobilised proximally to permit the whole segment being slid forward. It can survive as an island and be shifted distally for about 1 cm (Fig. 2.2D).

(b) *Base of the index and middle fingers as an ulnar flap.* A rotation flap based on the ulnar side (Fig. 2.8B) can be developed from the skin at the base of the middle and index fingers including the common digital branches of the median nerve to provide sensitive skin over the middle finger stump or the central area of the degloved metacarpal hand. Sensation over the radial aspect of the index finger can be preserved by leaving the most radial common digital branch of this region untouched in the transfer. Alternatively sensation over this region may be restored by another rotation flap from the radial innervated dorsal skin over the 2nd metacarpal and base of the index finger if such is available.

If needed, the ulnar innervated skin can be separated from this palmar flap to be utilised over the little finger remnants (Fig. 2.10). The distal part of these median and ulnar inner-

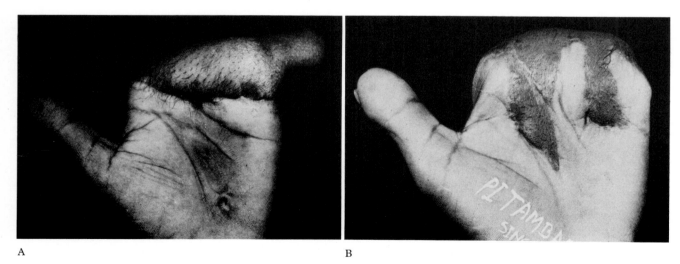

A   B

Figure 2.10
A and B, Show the possible use of the palmar skin at three strategic areas of grasp.

vated segments could still be converted into island flaps for further advancement and adjustment for longer stumps.

(c) *Base of the middle/ring fingers as a radial flap (Fig. 2.6C).* A flap could also be developed based radially on the neurovascular bundles and their cutaneous twigs supplying the skin over the base of the ring and middle fingers. This will supply the innervated skin over the strategic area on the palmar and radial aspects of the index finger stump. The three common digital branches of the median nerve are retained with the flap (Fig. 2.11A, B and C). The distal part of such a flap could also

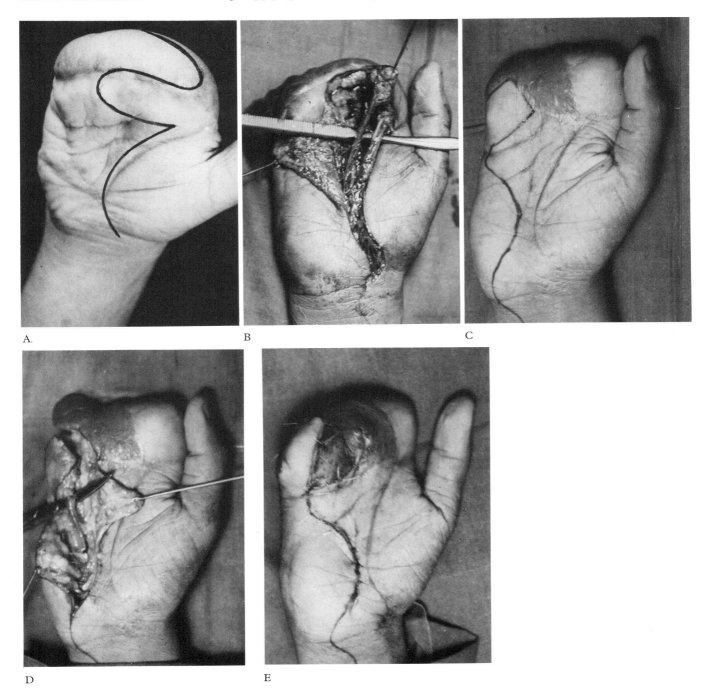

A.

B.

C.

D

E

Figure 2.11
A–E, Illustrate the technique of rotation advancement on neurovascular pedicles of the radially based median flap for index finger stump and ulnar innervated flap for little finger stump.

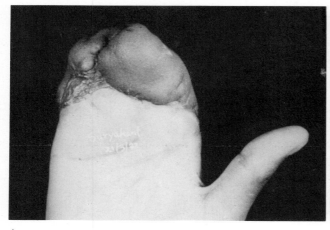

A

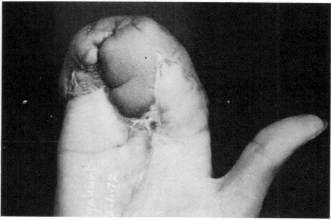

B

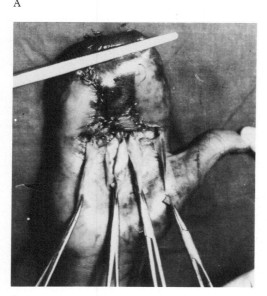

C

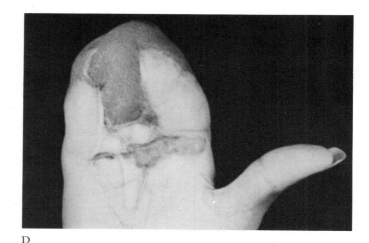

D

Figure 2.12
Illustrates the possible conversion of the median and ulnar flaps into islands for further advancement and adjustment on longer stumps.
A, Initial coverage by pedicled flap skin.
B, Rotation advancement achieved by radial based median flap and ulnar innervated flap.
C, Mobilisation of the distal portion of these flaps on neurovascular bundles.
D, Final advancement achieved.

be converted into a creeping type of island (Fig. 2.12) for further advancement on longer stumps.

(d) *Ulnar innervated segment of the palm (Fig. 2.8D)*. This is based on the digital nerves and vessels of the little finger and ulnar neurovascular bundles of the ring finger supplying the ulnar third of the palm. The area of the flap usually developed is distal to the proximal palmar crease and includes the digital branches of the ulnar nerve. This is suitable for migration to supply sensitive skin over the remains of the little finger or a reconstructed ulnar post in a metacarpal hand (Fig. 2.11 C, D and E).

The technique of raising these two last described flaps is illustrated in Figures 2.11 and 2.12 which are self-explanatory regarding the incisions, dissections and possible advancement achieved by these flaps. The flaps could be designed as 'Z' plasty flaps taking advantage of the loose pedicle grafted skin over the stumps which is used to fit into the defects created at the donor sites and obviates the necessity of free grafts. The method combines the principles of transposition, rotation and advancement on neurovascular pedicles to obtain the maximum sensation in hard pressed circumstances. The neurovascular attachments may limit the advancement initially due to tension imposed on them, but this is not a handicap as their inclusion allows the conversion of distal parts of the flaps into islands of sensory skin for final adjustment or for further advancement over the longer stumps.

The advancement of these flaps is limited to 2·5 to 3 cm. They are well suited to provide sensory cover over the proximal phalanges. This is best achieved by mobilisation of the specific neurovascular bundles proximally and requires dissection of the palmar fascia and its septa up to the wrist and undermining of the flaps keeping the nerves and vessels entering the flap intact. Sensation is never lost after such transfers though it may initially be diminished owing to stretching of the nerves. It usually takes 9 to 12 weeks for the flaps to recover their initial sensation. The grade of sensation achieved is that of tactile gnosis. The benefit of these operations is well appreciated by the patient as may be judged by their agreeing to undergo surgery in multiple stages. For sensory rehabilitation of the degloved mutilated hand, multiple stage operations are unavoidable as failure will add further insult. The creeping method of advancement assures safety in scarcity conditions. With a little ingenuity many of these flaps can find their use in osteoplastic reconstructive surgery of the mutilated hand.

ACKNOWLEDGEMENT

Figures 2.1, 2.4, 2.5, 2.8, 2.9, 2.10, 2.11 and 2.12 are reprinted from *Hand*, (1974) Journal of the British Society for Surgery of the Hand, **6**, No. 3, 247–254, with the kind permission of the Editor.

BIBLIOGRAPHY

ADAMSON, J. E., HORTON, C. E. & CRAWFORD, H. H. (1967). Sensory rehabilitation of the injured thumb. *Plastic and Reconstructive Surgery*, **40**, 53.

BOYES, J. H. (1964). In *Bunnell's Surgery of the Hand*, 4th Edition, p. 190. Philadelphia: M. B. Lippincott Company.

BRAILLER, F. & HORNER, R. L. (1960). Sensory cross finger pedicle graft. *Journal of Bone and Joint Surgery*, **51A**, 1264–1268.

CAUL, J. S. Jr. (1969). Radial innervated cross finger flap. *Journal of Bone and Joint Surgery*, **51A**, 1257–1263.

HOLEVICH, J. (1963). A new method of restoring sensibility to the thumb. *Journal of Bone and Joint Surgery*, **45B**, 496–502.

HUESTON, J. (1966). Local flap repair of fingertip injuries. *Plastic and Reconstructive Surgery*, **37**, 349–350.

JOSHI, B. B. (1970). One-stage repair for distal amputation of the thumb. *Plastic and Reconstructive Surgery*, **45**, 613–615.

JOSHI, B. B. (1972). Dorsolateral flap from same finger to relieve flexion contracture. *Plastic and Reconstructive Surgery*, **49**, 186–189.

JOSHI, B. B. (1974). A local dorso-lateral island flap for restoration of sensation after avulsion injury of finger tip pulp. *Plastic and Reconstructive Surgery*, **54**, 175–182.

LITTLER, J. W. (1959). *Neurovascular Skin Island Transfer in Reconstructive Hand Surgery*, ed. Wallace, A. B. p. 175. Transactions of the International Society of Plastic Surgeons Second Congress, London. Edinburgh: E. & S., Livingstone Ltd.

MOBERG, E. (1958). Objective method for determining the functional value of sensibility in the hand. *Journal of Bone and Joint Surgery*, **40B**, 454–476.

MILFORD, L. (1971). The hand, one of the volumes in *Campbell's Operative Orthopaedics*, 5th Edition, pp. 8 and 11, ed. Crenshaw, A. H. St Louis: C. V. Mosby.

NICOLLE, F. V. & WOLHOUSE, F. M. (1966). Restoration of sensory function in severe degloving injuries of the hand. *Journal of Bone and Joint Surgery*, **48A**, 1511–1518.

O'BRIEN, B. McC. (1968). Neurovascular island pedicle flaps for terminal amputations and digital scars. *British Journal of Plastic Surgery*, **21**, 259–261.

TUBIANA, R. & DUPARC, J. (1961). Restoration of sensibility in the hand by neurovascular skin island transfer. *Journal of Bone and Joint Surgery*, **43B**, 474–480.

WILSON, J. N. (1964). Restoration of sensation by neurovascular pedicle skin graft. *Journal of Bone and Joint Surgery*, **46A**, 216.

3. DIGITAL REPLANTATION

B. McC. O'Brien, A. M. MacLeod and W. A. Morrison

Amputated digits are now being replanted with increasing frequency. Though the initial survival of the part is dependent upon the patency of the microvascular anastomoses, the resultant function depends upon the adequacy of the nerve, tendon and bone union. Hence the decision to re-attach an amputated part must be made with a knowledge of the likely outcome of the various repairs.

INDICATIONS FOR DIGITAL REPLANTATION

In the hand which has suffered multiple injuries, all parts which can be expected to regain some function should be replaced (O'Brien and MacLeod, 1975). This decision to replant is often not made until all structures have been identified and the extent of the damage recognised clearly. Amputated thumbs are always replanted if possible, but a decision to replant a single, completely amputated finger, including the index, requires a special circumstance in an adult. Three months may be needed to regain useful function. Manual labour is impossible in the adult during this period, and the pattern of activity becomes so fixed that even when the single digit could be used it is ignored. Some women strongly request replantation of a single digit as they consider the loss of a finger to be a considerable cosmetic deformity. They will persevere with rehabilitation particularly if there is little economic loss. In a child, any part that can be repaired should be replanted, as the good results of tendon and nerve surgery, combined with high quality healing of the wound in children, make all the replanted parts useful.

Replantation requires careful consideration of the patient's age, occupation, dominance of the hand and the overall attitude and wishes of the patient. Guillotine amputations and those with only moderate crushing give the best chance of survival. Moderate crush injuries have formed the largest group and, whether completely or incompletely amputated, 80 to 90 per cent have survived. Avulsion injuries present considerable problems and only a few successful replantations have been achieved, but no attempt should be made if the vessels are torn out at a very distal level. It is recommended that only avulsed thumbs should be replanted and in these, early repair of the arteries is preferred, often with long microvenous grafts. Gross avulsion of nerves or tendons may preclude replantation (Fig. 3.1).

Amputated digits with gross crushing, much tissue loss, extensive vessel damage or multiple fractures, are not suitable for replantation.

A unique opportunity for improvisation exists in multiple amputations when the least damaged amputated part may be replanted on the most useful stump, to provide a digit with better function than would be the case were the replantations made in their true positions. It is better to obtain one finger functioning well in an optimal site than to have two less functional digits (Fig. 3.2). The Sixth People's Hospital, Shanghai (1973), replanted 13 grossly damaged fingers, with digital transpositions, 9 of which were successful.

For multiple replantations, at least two trained surgeons are recommended, to reduce operating time and enable as much primary surgery as possible to be carried out.

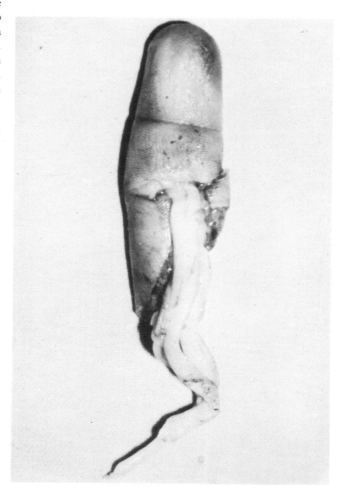

Figure 3.1
Avulsed digit which is unsuitable for replantation.

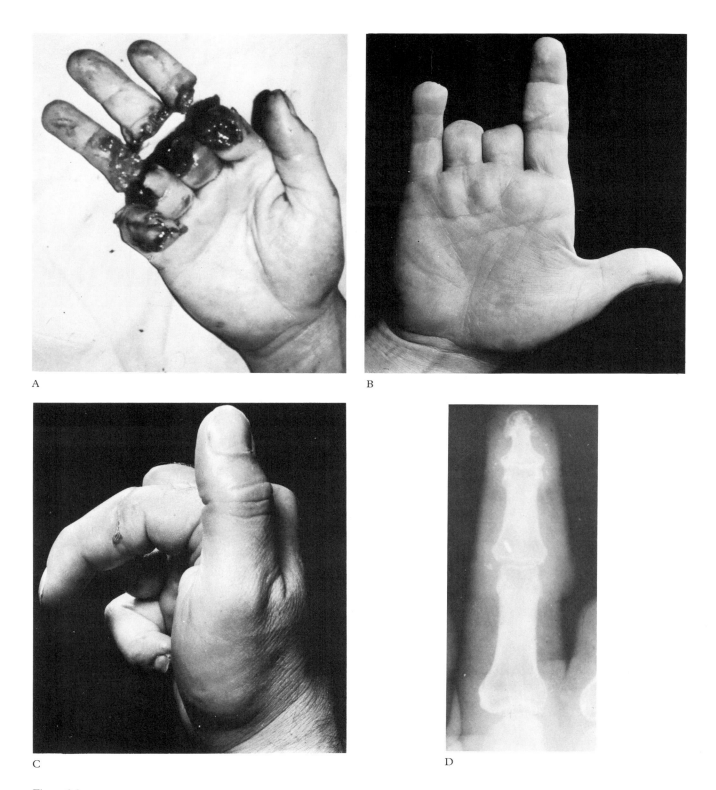

Figure 3.2
A, Saw cut amputations of the index, middle and ring fingers in a 29-year-old man.
B, Replantation of the middle finger on the index finger stump at the proximal interphalangeal joint level, retaining the articular surface of each digit. Seen at 4 months.
C, Flexion of the same finger at 4 months.
D, X-ray of the same replanted middle finger on the index stump at 4 months. The level of replantation was at the proximal interphalangeal joint level.

C

PREOPERATIVE MANAGEMENT IN DIGITAL REPLANTATION

FIRST AID

Some knowledge of the achievements of modern microsurgical techniques by the attending medical officer, ambulance attendant and the general public is essential to prevent the tragic loss, through ignorance, of a unique opportunity to re-attach amputated parts. In addition, it should also be remembered that a part, so irreversibly damaged that it cannot be replaced in its usual situation, can be valuable as a donor of tissues to another partly damaged area in the same patient.

The replanted fingers have been retrieved from many sources including machines, factory floors, fields, garbage tins and even a compost heap. The longest time before commencement of surgery has been 8 hours after injury. The ischaemic time for digital replantation is not as crucial or as serious as for major replantation, due to the absence of muscle in the replant and the ease of cooling. The severed part is placed in a clean plastic bag within a container of ice, to cool the part without freezing it. In the absence of a plastic bag, a moistened towel completely isolating the tissue from direct contact with the ice, may be used.

If gross organic contamination of amputated tissue has occurred, it is reasonable to irrigate the tissue gently with water from a tap. Normally this is not required and the tissue should, in no circumstances be placed in fluid, particularly antiseptics, which can cause cellular damage. Tissues should not be removed from a specimen however damaged it may appear.

A sterile dressing covers the stump and, for an incomplete amputation, a simple splint immobilises the limb to prevent kinking of any intact vessels. A tourniquet should not be used at this stage. On rare occasions, it may be necessary to apply an arterial clamp carefully to the very end of a vessel to arrest bleeding, reducing to a minimum the loss of vascular tissue. The clamp should not be left hanging unsupported from the wound, as this will inevitably cause further damage to the vessel. All tissue is carefully collected and a check made that all amputated parts have been recovered. This early management and the role of the ambulance officer, have been described (O'Brien and Haw, 1976).

If the general condition of the patient is satisfactory, arrangements are made for his rapid transportation to the nearest microsurgery centre. Transportation by air is preferable for journeys beyond 150 km (93 miles). The centre should be contacted as soon as possible after the injury and details of initial management, cause of injury and subsequent transfer, discussed with the surgical staff. The operating theatre can then be warned in advance and the required number of specialist surgeons assembled.

CASUALTY TREATMENT

Cooling of the amputated extremity is continued whilst an assessment of the local and general condition is made. Blood transfusion is sometimes required and a photographic record made. X-rays are taken of the stump and severed part to determine the injury level, and if any further bony damage is present at a lower level. Antibiotics are commenced and repeated 4 hourly. Prophylactic measures against tetanus are taken.

TECHNIQUE

The detailed operative technique of microvascular surgery as applied to replantation has previously been described (O'Brien et al., 1973; O'Brien, 1976).

Thorough cleansing and débridement are performed, the appropriate structures for repair are identified and the adequacy of the proximal arterial flow determined. Vein grafts may be used to bridge any gap following proximal vessel resection, especially for avulsion amputations. A tourniquet is useful during identification of structures and sometimes during repair of the vessels. In multiple replantations the tourniquet can be re-applied after revascularisation of the first digit.

An occasional digital amputation will be inoperable on account of damage to, or because of, inadequately sized veins. In four cases, no revascularisation was achieved primarily and replantation did not proceed any further, the digits being removed. Bone shortening by 0·5 to 1 cm is usually necessary to allow easy approximation of skin and repair of other tissues, particularly nerves, without tension. Oblique Kirschner pins usually suffice for fixation.

Unless the period of ischaemia without cooling has been unduly long in digital amputations, the arterial anastomosis is not performed until the other structures have been repaired. All the dorsal structures are repaired first and the skin closed before commencing the volar surgery. Care is taken to ligate superfluous veins at the wound edges as heparinisation later will lead to severe bleeding in the postoperative stage. At least two veins should be anastomosed and more, if easily found. Preferably, two arteries are joined to increase security against arterial thrombosis which has been the main cause of failure.

Emphasis is placed on careful primary repair of flexor tendons. Any secondary surgery is rendered difficult by excessive scar tissue and the dissection may threaten the integrity of the repaired vessels and nerves. Resection of flexor tendons followed by the insertion of a silastic rod may be considered primarily if good skin cover can be assured.

Simple capsular repairs are performed in amputations through joints but formal arthrodeses are only occasionally made primarily.

Illustrative cases are shown in Figures 3.3 and 3.4.

POSTOPERATIVE MANAGEMENT

The uncomplicated microvascular replant requires the minimum of postoperative care. Regular observations are made by the medical and nursing staff of the warmth of the digit, its colour and the capillary return which is the most important index of the circulation. Nurses vary in their assessment of colour changes in microvascular replants, and their task is more difficult with poor illumination at night.

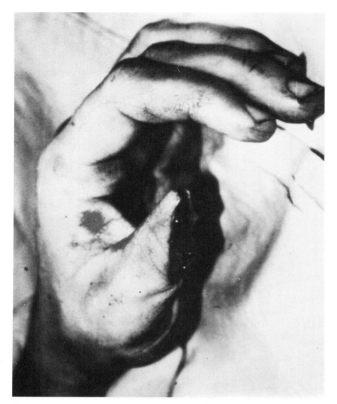

A

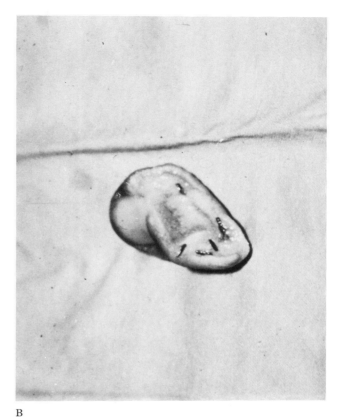

B

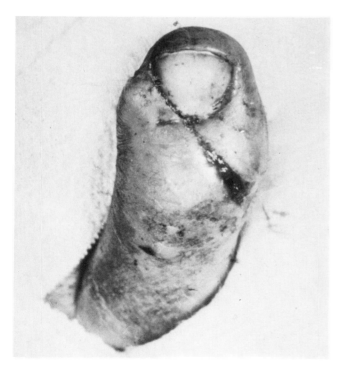

C

Figure 3.3
A, Oblique amputation of the distal left thumb.
B, Amputated distal thumb of the same patient. Clips might be in the vessels.
C, Replantation of the severed thumb which involved microvenous graft of the radial digital artery and two dorsal veins.

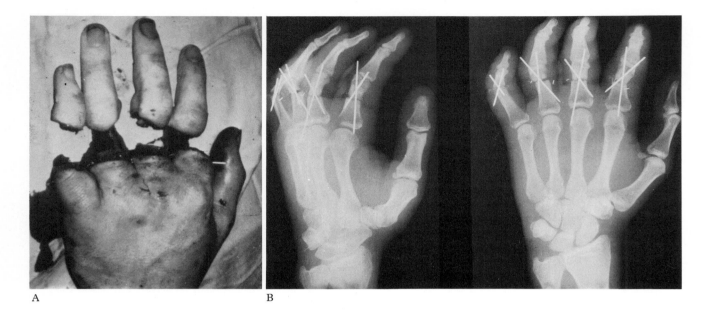

A   B

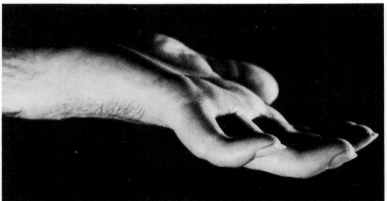

C

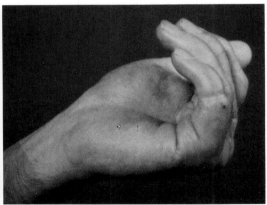

D

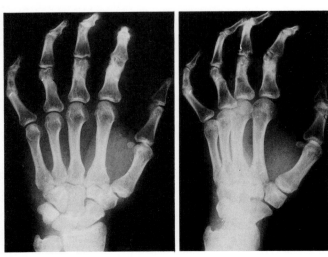

E

Figure 3.4
A, Saw cut amputations of the four fingers in a young man through the proximal phalanges.
B, Early postoperative X-ray of the same patient with satisfactory skeletal fixation.
C, Successful replantation of four fingers with total primary reconstruction after 1 year.
D, Flexion of the replanted fingers at 1 year.
E, X-rays of the same replanted fingers at 1 year.

Colour changes in darkly pigmented races such as the negro, are frequently of little or no help, and here the colour of the nail bed should be closely inspected.

The authors have not felt the need for Doppler machines to follow the circulatory state except in isolated instances, and believe that these aids are of minor importance compared with the standard clinical signs.

The temperature of replanted digits is a reliable index of the total blood flow in the digit. Any interruption of blood flow to the digit is followed rapidly by a drop in temperature of the avascular part. Manipulation is kept to a minimum, and the dressing is not changed for several days. No constricting blood clots or dressings are permitted, as these can interfere with venous return.

The arm is elevated above the level of the shoulder for at least 10 days to counteract the swelling due to interference with lymphatic drainage. Excessive elevation of the limb may lead to a decreased arterial inflow and thrombosis. The posture is changed to vary arterial or venous flow as parameters dictate. A hypotensive episode may also precipitate thrombosis. Usually the digit is pinker and warmer than normal for the first 2 to 3 days, with a brisk capillary return. An adequate blood level should be maintained. 1 000 000 u of penicillin and 0·5 g of ampicillin are given intravenously, four times daily and smoking is not permitted.

ANTICOAGULANTS

Anticoagulants are deferred for 24 hours to allow the wounds to seal. The present regimen consists of aspirin 1 g daily and persantin (Dipyridamole) 25 mg four times daily given orally and commenced after surgery, to reduce the adhesiveness of platelets and to lower plasma fibrinogen. Macrodex, 6 per cent, 500 ml in 4 hours, is given immediately after operation and on the second and third days for its platelet effect.

Heparin, 5000 u intravenously as a starting dose, is commenced 24 hours postoperatively, followed by 25 000 to 30 000 u in 1 litre of dextrose in isotonic saline given intravenously via a paediatric burette during the next 24 hours. The daily clotting time is maintained at 25 to 30 minutes and stability should be reached within 24 hours. The Kaolin-partial thromboplastin time, a more precise measurement, is determined every second day and should be above 55 seconds. Heparin is considered to be the most important single anticoagulant but it is not used for amputations proximal to the necks of the metacarpals as the vessels at that level are adequate in size and, moreover, bleeding muscle masses can lead to haematoma formation.

Intravenous therapy is discontinued after 12 days as no digital loss has occurred beyond this period. Aspirin and persantin are maintained for another week.

COMPLICATIONS

SWELLING

This occurs in every case but is minimal if there is adequate venous drainage. Tight sutures are released and in only two patients was a dorsal decompression necessary to improve circulation.

VENOUS CONGESTION

This is recognised by a drop in the temperature of the part and a flushed, purple appearance associated with a very rapid capillary return. In the early stages of venous congestion, the colour of the microvascular replant may show little change but the very brisk capillary return is a warning signal. The pulp of a congested digit has an increased turgor and a feeling of fullness.

The replant is inspected for constricting bandages, tight sutures or haematomas. Suspect sutures should be removed and additional elevation employed. Gentle milking along the dorsum of the digit towards the microvenous anastomoses, may occasionally dislodge a loosely adherent thrombus and improve the venous outflow. Incisions in the distal pulp confirm the diagnosis and can improve the colour of the digit.

The anticoagulation level should be checked and adjusted accordingly. If indicated, 6 per cent macrodex can be resumed. If there is no response in 3 to 4 hours to these conservative measures, then reoperation is desirable and the anticoagulant therapy is discontinued. Reoperation must not be delayed as secondary thrombosis of the arterial anastomosis can result. Venous thrombosis has been seen within the first 10 days on six occasions and one case was successful on reoperation.

ARTERIAL OCCLUSION

This is the commonest cause of failure and Tsai (1975) has confirmed this in his series. The first sign of arterial insufficiency is a slowed capillary return and this slowing becomes more marked as the vascular inflow becomes progressively impaired. The colour of the replant becomes a bluish mottled white, the temperature of the replant has decreased and the pulp has an empty feel. Thrombosis has developed as early as a few hours and as late as 12 days.

Again, constricting bandages, tight sutures and accumulation of haematoma should be released, although these factors are seldom a source of arterial insufficiency. An adverse level of anticoagulation should be corrected. Lowering of the replant below heart level may be of some value, but a careful watch must be kept for signs of venous congestion or failure of the arterial input to improve. Minor arterial insufficiency may improve spontaneously due to dissolution of thrombus or relief of spasm. Early surgical intervention is usually the best course.

REVISIONARY SURGERY

Revisionary surgery to alleviate deficiency in circulation is difficult. Anastomosis of unused vessels is more reliable than further surgery to the original anastomosis as the friable vessels are difficult to resuture and the intimal changes which occur in association with thrombosis predispose to further clotting. If no alternative vessels are available, then the faulty anastomosis should be resected and a vein graft interposed. Vein grafts are readily obtained from the volar aspect of the forearm and should be placed under a little tension to avoid kinking and rotation, on the establishment of the blood flow.

POSTOPERATIVE BLEEDING

This results from failure to coagulate or clip unsatisfied veins and occasionally from a small hole at the arterial anastomosis. Considerable transfusion may be needed. The bleeding occurs when the circulation in the finger appears adequate. During reoperation, healing wounds are disrupted with a loss of early peripheral circulation. Even though the bleeding area is brought under control, arterial thrombosis can occur during the operation and, despite revisional vascular surgery, circulation may not be adequately established. Conservative measures give the finger an equal, or better, chance than reoperation. Hence it is recommended that heparinisation be discontinued and the circulation of the digit observed closely.

INFECTION

Infection has been seen in only two cases despite the fact that the digits have been retrieved from many dirty places.

SKIN NECROSIS

Occasionally some skin necrosis is seen, usually on the dorsal surface. If this overlies the vein anastomosis, there is a high risk of thrombosis. The skin necrosis is treated conservatively unless there is clear evidence of vascular impairment in which case the necrotic skin should be excised and a vein graft, or venous pedicle, from an adjacent digit or dorsum of the hand, used. A split thickness skin graft or local flap covers the vessel. If the circulation is not impaired, the skin is removed gradually after 2 weeks. Any thrombosed vein underneath the skin necrosis may not need further surgery if the circulation of the digit has remained satisfactory.

BONY NON-UNION

One case of bony non-union has been observed at the base of the proximal phalanx of the thumb, but this acts as a pseudo-joint and does not seriously impair function. It is thus an uncommon complication but adequate primary skeletal fixation is stressed.

SECONDARY RECONSTRUCTION

Dense scar at the replantation site is a strong argument for primary reconstruction in an effort to avoid secondary surgery. If there is doubt about the circulation of the finger at the primary stage, the repair of tendons and nerves may be deferred. It is usually possible to achieve the repair of the digital nerve adjacent to the digital arterial repair, thus avoiding exposure of this area at a later date with possible damage to the repaired artery.

Silicone rods are used for two-stage flexor tendon grafting. Occasionally they can be inserted primarily to avoid closure of the thecal tunnel, replacing them at about 2 months with tendon grafting. Silastic joints have been used in one patient in this series and Lindsay (1972) has inserted a silicone joint into the metacarpophalangeal joint of a replanted thumb.

RESULTS

These are summarised in Tables 3.1 to 3.3, and comprise 103 digits in 74 cases. Of 55 complete amputations, 38 (68 per cent) have survived and this series incorporates all cases including the one failure before the first successful case. There were 47 incomplete amputations with 38 survivals (81 per cent). The ages of the patients ranged from 13 months to 70 years, and the level of amputation from the metacarpophalangeal joints to the distal interphalangeal joints. Of the 38 successful replantations of completely amputated digits, 9 survivals out of 11 (81 per cent) were guillotine injuries, and 26 out of 28 (93 per cent) were localised crush injuries. Only 3 of 16 diffusely crushed, or avulsed, digits survived. Of 32 localised crush incomplete amputations, 30 (94 per cent) survived and of the 15 avulsion and diffuse crush incomplete group, 8 survived (53 per cent). An incomplete amputation was considered to be an ischaemic compound injury of a digit with division of bone, tendons and nerves, and sometimes, the management of this injury can be more difficult than a complete amputation. If the avulsion group is excluded, 90 per cent of the complete amputations in the guillotine and localised crush groups survived and 94 per cent in the incomplete amputations. In the avulsion and/or diffuse crush groups, only 18 per cent of the complete amputations survived

TABLE 3.1 This series covers all cases including the one failure before the first successful case

Results of amputated digits	
Cases	74
Amputated digits	103
Complete amputations	55
Survival	38 (68%)
Incomplete amputations	47
Survival	38 (81%)

TABLE 3.2 Analysis of digital replantations

		Nature of injury	Number	Survival	Total
Complete amputations	55	Guillotine	11	9	38
		Localised crush	28	26	
		Avulsion	16	3	
Incomplete amputations	47	Localised crush	32	30	38
		Avulsion and/or			
		Diffuse crush	15	8	

TABLE 3.3 Survival: digital replantation

Guillotine and localised moderate crush	Complete 90%	Incomplete 94%
Avulsion and/or diffuse crush	Complete 18%	Incomplete 53%

and 53 per cent of the incomplete group. Most of the avulsed digits required reoperation, constituting approximately 80 per cent of the reoperations.

LONG-TERM FUNCTION

Long-term follow-up has extended to 6 years. Improvement has been observed up to 3 years. There have been only ten requests for late amputation of any digit. In some cases the patient depends almost entirely on his replanted digit or digits for useful function of the hand.

SENSATION

Following primary digital nerve repair, the result of two-point discrimination has ranged from 3 to 20 mm, with the greater majority at a level below 10 mm (Morrison *et al.*, 1975). These levels are comparable with those obtained following simple nerve injuries. In a 60-year-old man with a four finger replantation, a 4 mm two-point discrimination at the tips of all fingers was obtained. In some cases unpleasant hyperaesthesia has interfered with the function of the replanted digit and amputation was performed. The long duration of ischaemia observed in several fingers has not affected the eventual quality of nerve regeneration. The value of accurate nerve repairs cannot be over-emphasised as most of the worthwhile function of the surviving digits will depend on their sensibility. If the nerves are not repaired primarily, the retraction of the nerve in dense scar tissue leaves a defect that requires subsequent nerve grafting in difficult surgical conditions with danger to a previously repaired digital artery essential to the survival of the digit. A nerve graft bypassing the site of anastomosis can lessen this risk.

MOTOR FUNCTION

All the patients, except the two requiring amputation have benefited from their final range of motion, even though it has been restricted in all but a few. Of three, four-finger replantations, two have gained a worthwhile range of motion, but one poorly motivated patient has not achieved a satisfactory result despite two-stage flexor tendon grafts. Primary arthrodesis in a satisfactory position may be performed if the level of amputation is at the proximal interphalangeal joint. The power of the digit may be augmented by tenodesis, e.g. at the distal interphalangeal joint. Tenolysis has only occasionally been performed although Ch'en (1972) advises it in many cases. Every effort should be made to obtain a high quality primary repair of the flexor profundus tendon.

GROWTH

All the replanted digits show some permanent degree of atrophy and are shorter. Nail growth has been observed to be more rapid than normal in some replanted digits and also harder. Provided the epiphysis is undamaged, digits in children are growing within normal limits, allowing for the original bone shortening.

OTHER FEATURES

The many variables render an objective assessment of the function of the replanted parts difficult and furthermore such assessment would not be a true indication of the usefulness of the part. However, all patients have been carefully followed up and are seen to be using the affected fingers and hands. Many patients have returned to occupations requiring manual dexterity and strength. Subjectively there has been a high level of success.

In multiple amputations, a surgical team with at least two surgeons and two assistants, and supporting trained operating room nursing staff, is preferred. An active microsurgical research programme is an advantage in training personnel and an adequate experience in hand surgery is vital. Every large city should have one centre equipped to deal with this type of hand injury. It is important that work be made available to patients early in their rehabilitation, so that a high level of morale is achieved. Tools at their work may need modification. The higher the level of motivation the better the final, functional results. Satisfactory final results have been achieved in most patients but continuing evaluation is required. The usefulness of replanted digits is superior to prostheses and these parts have required less rehabilitation than the unamputated digits which have suffered severe crushing or burning injuries.

CONCLUSION

The revascularisation of completely or incompletely amputated digits can be achieved by careful attention to established microvascular techniques and is a rewarding procedure if reasonable case selection is performed. It is important to aim for good function rather than mere survival of the part, but extreme care is required in any revisionary or secondary surgery.

BIBLIOGRAPHY

LINDSAY, W. R. N. (1972). Personal communication.
MORRISON, W. A., O'BRIEN, B. McC., MACLEOD, A. M. & NEWING, R. K. (1975). Long term nerve function in replantation surgery of the hand and digits. *Annales de Chirurgie*, **29**, 1041–1045.
O'BRIEN, B. McC., MACLEOD, A. M., MILLER, G. D. H., NEWING, R. K., HAYHURST, J. W. & MORRISON, W. A. (1973). Clinical replantation of digits. *Plastic and Reconstructive Surgery*, **52**, 491–502.
O'BRIEN, B. McC. & MACLEOD, A. M. (1975). Replantation surgery. *Transactions of the Sixth International Congress of Plastic and Reconstructive Surgery*, Paris. In press.
O'BRIEN, B. McC. & HAW, C. S. (1976). Microsurgical reattachment of traumatic amputations: the role of the ambulance officer. *Journal of the Institute of Ambulance Officers* (Australia), **1**, 2–4.
O'BRIEN, B. McC. (1977). *Microvascular Reconstructive Surgery*, Edinburgh: Churchill Livingstone.
SIXTH PEOPLE'S HOSPITAL, SHANGHAI (1973). Replantation of severed limbs and fingers. *Chinese Medical Journal*, **1**, 3–10.
TSAI, TSE-MIN (1975). Experimental and clinical application of microvascular surgery. *Annals of Surgery*, **2**, 169–177.

4. *FINGER-TIP AMPUTATION*

J. Glicenstein

The prime object in the treatment of finger-tip amputations is to provide a finger end with skin of good sensibility and to reduce its tactile deficiency as much as possible. Only the highly differentiated skin of the volar aspect of the finger can match in quality that of the missing pulp.

Wherever possible, the amputated extremity must be made good by this skin.

IMMEDIATE REPAIR

METHODS

1. *Spontaneous healing by epithelialisation* (Vilain and Michon, 1968) is not the simplest form of treatment because it requires regular supervision of the patient for 3 to 6 weeks:
   The wound is covered with a non-adherent dressing (tulle gras or balsam of Peru)
   Progressive healing occurs with contraction at the edges and marginal epithelialisation (Fig. 4.1)

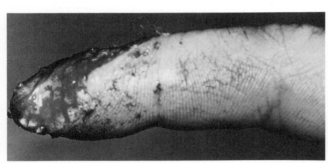

A

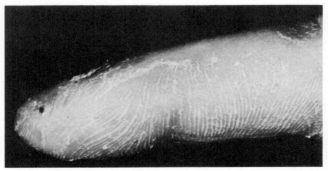

B

Figure 4.1
Spontaneous healing.
A, Tissue loss on sides and dorsum.
B, Condition at 3 weeks.

The finger-tip may become perfectly curved provided the amputation does not expose the terminal phalanx. Should bone be exposed, however, the scar may be adherent to it.

2. In distal loss on the dorsal aspect, excision of triangles of skin on either side facilitates simple closure of the finger end; similarly, shortening the bone by a few millimetres may, in certain cases, assist skin closure.

3. The application of a thin skin graft has two advantages; the skin takes well even on bone, healing taking about 10 days; shrinkage of such grafts is an important factor in spreading the skin of the pulp (Fig. 4.2).

4. Full thickness grafts, on the other hand, have virtually no place in the treatment of finger tip amputations except, possibly, for narrow defects on the sides. In fact, even at best, they provide rather a poor 'patch' lacking sensation (Fig. 4.3). However, Maquieira (1974) has recently advocated use of a full thickness graft together with the nerve supplying it suturing the latter to a sensory nerve at the recipient site.

5. When the amputated portion has been saved, should it be re-attached? We have all tried this and have had what appeared to have been successes from time to time. On

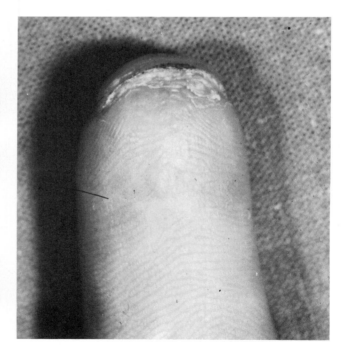

Figure 4.2
Thin skin graft drawn under the nail.

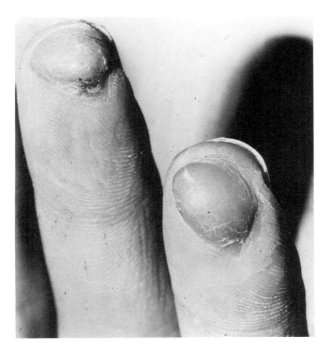

Figure 4.3
Full thickness grafts with ugly appearance and lacking sensibility.

removal of the eschar, the underlying pulp has healed spontaneously with shortening of the finger, this being quite obvious when comparing before and after photographs. Successful instances do, however, occur. Douglas (1959) has published 17 such but has also laid down very strict criteria when attempting this procedure:

Replacement within an hour of injury
Suturing with the aid of a loupe or microscope to obtain accurate matching of the finger prints

Re-attachment of the distal phalanx only after a clean cut amputation.

In these cases, sensory return is very rapid; 3 to 20 days. Apart from these ideal conditions it is better not to suture back the fragment in place unless it remains attached by a skin pedicle, however small.

6. A composite graft, the toe pulp graft advocated by McCash (1959) and by Marchac and Rousso (1971) should ensure a rapid return of sensation.

7. All the procedures so far described are suitable only for distal losses. When there is a major loss on the palmar aspect it is better to introduce a skin flap by a local plastic procedure. These local flaps are the most fascinating.

The Kutler procedure (Fischer, 1967) is very useful for distal slicing injuries. It involves advancing to the mid-line two lateral pulp flaps which retain their deep connections and closure of the secondary defects in V–Y manner. This is a safe flap and complications are rare, even in the hands of young surgeons (Fig. 4.4).

The palmar advancement flap of Moberg (1967) and Snow (1967) involves raising an extensive volar flap incorporating the neurovascular bundles. The flap is sutured to the end of the finger whilst the latter is flexed. Morel-Fatio and Nicoletis have made important criticisms of this procedure in that it damages the blood supply to the dorsum of the finger by dividing the dorsal branches of the digital arteries. A further proviso is that the procedure should only be attempted on fully mobile fingers.

A simpler and more certain method is the advancement-rotation flap of Hueston (1966) dissected superficial to one of the digital bundles whilst retaining the other in its base. The secondary defect is made good by a free graft (Fig. 4.5).

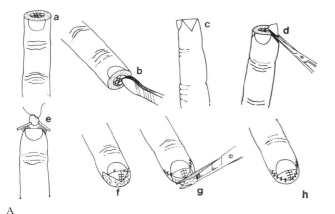

A

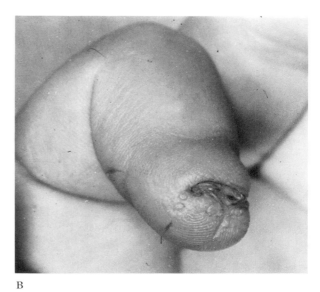

B

Figure 4.4
A, Kutler flap procedure. Technique (after Fischer, 1967). a, slicing injury; b, minimal trimming; c, outline of the two triangular flaps; d, minimal freeing; e, suture in midline; f, suture to nail; g, reduction of pulp; h, closure of tip.
B, Result of Kutler procedure.

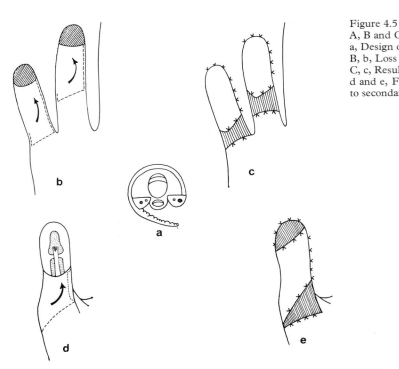

Figure 4.5
A, B and C Hueston flap.
a, Design of flap.
B, b, Loss of pulp.
C, c, Result of Hueston flaps.
d and e, Flap to cover exposed profundus tendon. Split skin grafts
to secondary defects.

A

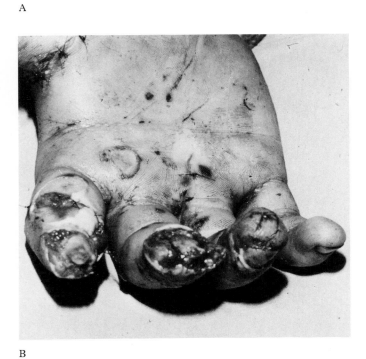

B

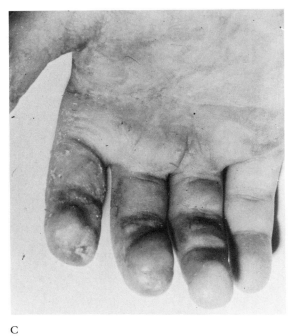

C

Innervated flaps of the Littler type have been advocated by Sullivan (1967) for emergency reconstruction of the thumb pulp. It would appear wiser to adopt a simpler form of treatment as a primary measure.

8. *Flaps from adjacent site.* There are few indications for these in the emergency treatment of amputated finger-tips. They are absolutely contra-indicated in cases of joint stiffness or in patients over 40 years of age. They can cause complica-

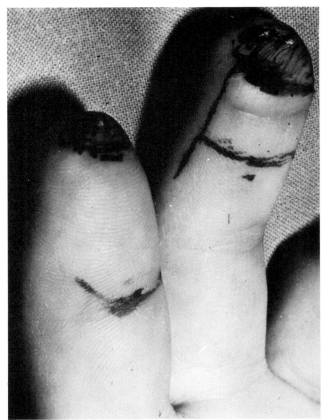

A

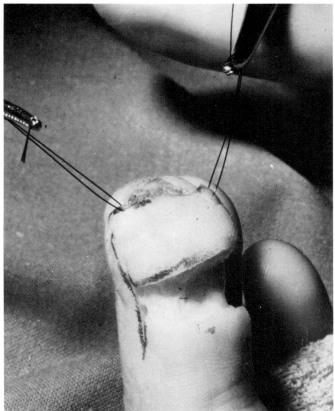

B

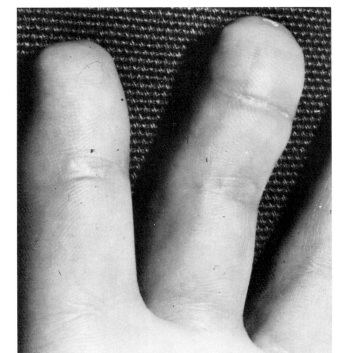

C

Figure 4.6
Milford flap (Milford, 1972) to repair defect on middle finger.
A, Design of flap. Note Hueston flap on index.
B, Neurovascular advancement flap.
C, Result: the distal scar on the middle finger-tip is similar to that which follows spontaneous healing following loss of finger-tip.

tions at the donor site. They may exaggerate in the mind of the manual worker the seriousness of an injury which requires more than one operation, but most important of all, they produce a 'blind pulp' which is slowly and poorly re-innervated. They may be useful, however, when extensive loss of substance largely denudes the phalanx. The classical techniques include the cross-finger flap and the thenar flap.

9. *Flaps from a distance*. These have no place in the treatment of amputations of the finger-tips.

INDICATIONS FOR VARIOUS TYPES OF TREATMENT

There is no one method suitable for every case. Considerable experience on the part of the surgeon is essential before embarking on a complicated flap. If the necessary surgical expertise is not available in such a case, it is better to cover the wound with a tulle gras dressing or apply a thin graft but the ideal is to carry out the definitive treatment immediately.

Each case is assessed on its merits and one must treat the amputation according to its level (distal or proximal), its direction (transverse, oblique either in a dorsal or palmar direction, radial or ulnar sides) whether a single or multiple digit injury.

1. *Distal amputations*: the simplest methods must always be used:

Loss of skin and pulp not involving bone are treated by tulle gras dressings or by excision of triangles of skin on either side in a dorsal slicing type of injury
Amputations through the tip of the terminal phalanx may be treated either by a thin split skin graft or a simple local flap procedure (Kutler type repair, for example).

2. Amputations through the base of the nail or a large pulp slicing injury present the most difficult problems. The Hueston flap is the most useful method.

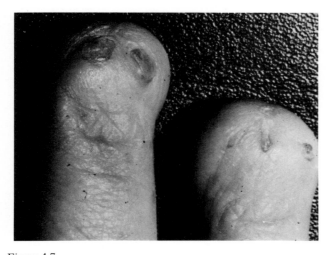

Figure 4.7
Nail remnants—clubbed finger.

3. Oblique amputations on either side may be treated by full thickness grafts.

4. Amputation of the distal phalanx of the thumb. It is only in such cases that the most complicated skin flaps should be considered (advancement of innervated flaps) but the Hueston flap is often useful.

In conclusion, the spontaneous re-epithelialisation and the dressing regime have their places. One must resist the temptation to undertake a delicate repair bearing in mind the disability period for the various methods as follows:

0 to 40 days for the tulle gras dressing regime or for spontaneous re-epithelialisation
2 months for a local skin flap (Kutler, Hueston)
4–6 months for a distant flap repair.

COMPLICATIONS FOLLOWING AMPUTATIONS OF FINGER-TIPS

These are numerous. They are often played down by the patients but may sometimes be troublesome and cause cosmetic disability.

1. Complications due to loss of pulp are seen particularly with the palmar slicing injuries. The finger end is shortened and adherent to bone. The use of an innervated advancement flap as advocated by Milford (1972) and Moberg (1967) provides an interesting solution to the problem (Fig. 4.6).

2. Nail complications are very frequent. When half of the nail is removed by amputation, it comes over the end of the stump and tends to grow in. It is troublesome and has an ugly appearance (Fig. 4.7). The setting back of the nail and its matrix results in a small but straighter nail. Nail remnants frequently persist and have to be removed with the residual part of the matrix (Fig. 4.8).

3. The clubbed finger-tip (Fig. 4.8A) is associated with loss of tissue at the end of the finger and presents a swollen pear-shaped appearance. Dufourmentel (1963) has described an elegant procedure for the correction of this deformity (Fig. 4.8B and C).

CONCLUSION

If one aims at restoring a perfect appearance in these injuries it is essential to manage the amputated finger-tip with extreme care and skill.

BIBLIOGRAPHY

ATASOY, E., IOAKIMIDIS, E., KASOAN, M., KURTZ, J. E. & KLEINERT, H. E. (1970). Reconstruction of amputated finger tip with tri-angular volar flap. *Journal of Bone and Joint Surgery*, **52A**, 921.
BOJSEN-MOILLIER, J., PERS, M. & SCHMIDT, A. (1961). Finger tip injuries: late results. *Acta chirurgica scandinavica*, **122**, 177.
DOUGLAS, B. (1959). Successful replacement of completely avulsed portions of fingers as composite grafts. *Plastic and Reconstructive Surgery*, **23**, 213.
DUFOURMENTEL, CL. (1963). Correction chirurgicale des extrémités digitales en 'massue'. *Annales de chirurgie plastique*, **8**, 99.

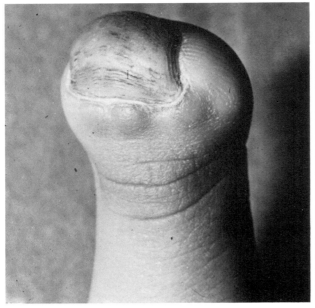

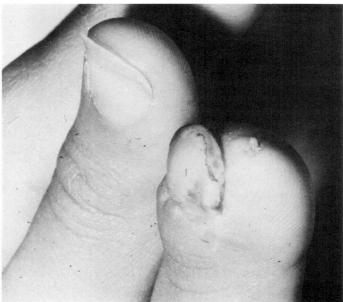

A   C

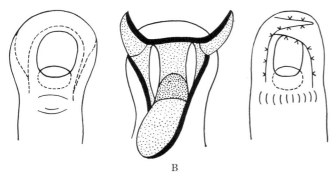

B

Figure 4.8
Parrot beak deformity.
A, Typical appearance with nail curved over finger-tip.
B, Correction of parrot beak deformity (Dufourmentel, 1963).
C, Result: a small nail remnant persists.

DUFOURMENTEL, CL., LOTTE, J. & ELBAZ, J. S. (1964). A propos de la réimplantation des extrémités digitales totalement détachées. *Annales de chirurgie plastique*, **9**, 165.

FISCHER, R. H. (1967). The Kutler method for repair of finger tip amputations. *Journal of Bone and Joint Surgery*, **49**, 317.

FLYNN, J. E. (1966). *Hand Surgery*. Baltimore: Williams and Wilkins.

GLICENSTEIN, J. (1971). Techniques de réparation des amputations des extrémités digitales. *Annales de chirurgie*, **25**, 1001.

GOSSET, J. & MICHON, J. (1967). Traitement des plaies fraîches de la main. *Rapport au 67e Congrès Français de Chirurgie*. Paris.

HUESTON, J. (1966). Local flap repair of finger tip injuries. *Plastic and Reconstructive Surgery*, **37**, 349.

ISELIN, M. F. (1967). *Traité de Chirurgie de la Main*. Paris, Ed. Méd. Flammarion.

KOMATSU, S. & TAMAI, S. (1968). Successful replantation of a completely cut-off thumb. *Plastic and Reconstructive Surgery*, **42**, 374.

McCASH, C. (1959). Toe pulp free grafts in finger-tips repair. *British Journal of Plastic Surgery*, **11**, 322.

MAQUIEIRA, N. O. (1974). An innervated full-thickness skin graft to restore sensibility to fingertips and heels. *Plastic and Reconstructive Surgery*, **53**, 568.

MARCHAC, D. & ROUSSO, M. (1971). La greffe cutanéopulpaire après amputation des extrémités digitales. *Annales de chirurgie plastique*, **17**, 51.

MICHON, J., DUFOURMENTEL, C., GLICENSTEIN, J., ROULLET, J. & VILAIN, R. (1970). Les amputations des extrémités digitales. *Annales de chirurgie plastique*, **15**, 277.

MILFORD, L. (1971). *The Hand*. From *Campbell's Operative Orthopaedics*, C. V. Mosby, 5th edition.

MOBERG, E. (1967). *Emergency Surgery of the Hand*. Edinburgh: Livingstone.

SNOW, J. W. (1967). The use of a volar flap for repair of fingertip amputations. A preliminary report. *Plastic and Reconstructive Surgery*, **40**, 163.

SULLIVAN, J. G., KELLEHER, J. C., BAIBAK, G. J., DEAN, R. K. & PINKNER, L. D. (1967). The primary application of an island flap in thumb and index finger injuries. *Plastic and Reconstructive Surgery*, **39**, 488.

VILAIN, R. & MICHON, J. (1968). *Chirurgie Plastique Cutanée de la Main chez l'Enfant et l'Adulte*. Paris: Masson.

5. MULTIPLE DIGIT AMPUTATIONS

J. Michon

Multiple amputations of the digits present many problems first and foremost being the nature of the primary procedure to be adopted in such a mutilating injury.

PRIMARY TREATMENT

We are all aware of the importance of the site of a wound and particularly in these injuries. Careful conservation of all viable tissue must be practised when undertaking débridement and bone removal kept to the absolute minimum. The soft tissue will be available at the time of wound closure when either a free graft or a local flap may be required. In the choice of procedure or the design of a local flap, the essential aim of tactile sensibility on the grasping surfaces must have first priority.

The second guiding principle in primary management is to make full use of what remains. If one has to amputate digits or digital remnants which cannot be saved, it is rare for one not to be able to make use of parts of them, for example skin, tendons, nerves or bone segments can often be used as free grafts, sometimes as pedicle transfers. This may allow one to conserve both tissue and function in the viable parts of the injured hand.

It is impossible, because of the wide individual variations from case to case, to make any further generalisations in this brief account, so much depends on one's experience and imaginative planning.

SECONDARY SURGICAL PROCEDURES

Following healing of a mutilating injury involving multiple amputations, a period of rehabilitation is necessary to restore suppleness and mobility to the remaining structures. One is now in a position to consider reconstructive procedures with restoration of grasping function in mind.

Paradoxically, it may sometimes be necessary to complete the removal of a part preserved at the initial procedure: such a finger conserved at the time of primary treatment may end up permanently stiff and painful and with trophic changes. This can have an adverse effect on the function of neighbouring digits which may be due to the linkage syndrome described by Verdan. The importance of this might easily be overlooked in these multiple digit amputations. Provided the metacarpal part of the hand is intact, two fingers separated by a gap from one another, provided they are functional, are just as useful as two fingers in close proximity. A single intact finger facing a mobile thumb also provides the hand with its essential function. In such a case, a rotation osteotomy through a metacarpal may improve both the pinch grip and the power grip particularly when the little finger is involved.

A single remaining finger may lack resistance against radial pressure of the thumb. The counter pressure for this is normally exerted by the first dorsal interosseous which stabilises the index finger. A tendon transfer to the radial interosseous can restore or re-inforce this function.

Finally, one can consider redistribution of the remaining fingers to improve prehension. Transfer of the index finger to the 3rd metacarpal increases the 1st web space in a remarkable way and improves the pinch grip. This procedure is particularly indicated if the thumb itself is short or lacks mobility.

6. SINGLE DIGIT AMPUTATIONS

J. Duparc, J-Y. Alnot and P. May

Mutilating injuries of the digits, excluding the thumb, constitute a group of defects which change or destroy the essential functions of the hand. Before considering the various aspects of finger amputations, it will be helpful to remind ourselves of prehensile function in the normal hand. We are then better able to understand the principles which govern restoration of prehension in the mutilated hand.

Prehension is achieved by a combination of power, sensibility and control of the hand by both the brain and the eyes.

In studying prehension we have considered four different grips which, though they concern the static phases of prehension, yet still enable one to make a sufficiently precise study of the various functions of the hand. These four grips are:

Digital pinch (thumb/fingers)
Palmar grip
Directional grip
Multiple pulp grip.

We shall stress the latter two which we consider very important in assessing the function both of the normal and of the mutilated hand.

1. *Digital pinch grip* (thumb, index, middle) (Fig. 6.1). These pinch grips with all their variations are essential, particularly the tip-to-tip pinch and the three-digit pinch (Fig. 6.2).

2. *The palmar grip* (Fig. 6.3) is at right angles to the axis of the hand often with ulnar deviation of the wrist which adds strength to the grip. This may be seen, for example, in the carrying of a suitcase.

3. *Directional grip* (Fig. 6.4A, B). This corresponds to the 'power grip' of Napier and Pulvertaft (1966) but seems to us to merit detailed study. In fact, each finger has a well-defined role to play. The index finger is the one with most directional function. The little finger ensures stability of the object and grips it. This directional grip is a combination of the two former grips and the degree of control of power and precision will depend on the position of the index finger. This is seen, for example, in the use of a screwdriver. The finger prints of the grasping areas may be demonstrated by using a screwdriver covered with powder (Fig. 6.4).

4. *Multiple pulp grip* (or spherical grip) (Fig. 6.5A, B). This corresponds to the 'precision grip' of Napier. This may be illustrated in the grasping of an electric light bulb and here again one may study the finger prints of the functional sites by using a bulb covered with powder.

Damage to these sites leads to altered function. When the hand has been mutilated, prehension is altered and the various grips described are modified.

Study of the four grips is of paramount importance in evaluating the effect of the mutilation and in deciding on the optimal level of amputation. However severe the injury, the surgeon's aim is to restore prehension and the most useful grip in as conservative a way as possible.

In each case one must consider two possibilities regarding treatment. One is shortening of the bone in order to achieve primary suture provided this be achieved without increasing the functional disability. The other is preserving the whole length of the bone by the use of a more or less complicated surgical reconstruction. One should try to avoid, at any price, a stump of a length which will not be functionally better than one obtained by shortening the bone. A clinical knowledge of alterations in grip related to the types of amputation enables one to choose the optimal level.

From a functional point of view, the problems vary according to which finger is damaged and also to the level of the injury.

Finally, one should bear in mind that adequate sensibility is necessary for fine manipulations. This involves co-ordination between the sensory impulses and the motor responses. Fingers lacking sensation or which are either painful or stiff, are rarely used.

For classification, we divide amputations into four groups:

Amputations of a single finger
Hemi-amputations
Sub-total amputations
Total amputations

SINGLE DIGIT AMPUTATIONS

Single digit amputations enable one to make very interesting observations of prehension. Alterations in the four grips may be accurately assessed and different cases compared. Amputations of the index finger are by far the most frequent.

We shall consider each of the four fingers in turn.

We divide each finger into zones depending on the amputation site and where problems presented by the stump are virtually identical. These zones are separated by levels which are not elective levels for amputation but rather border lines between two different types of stump. The definition of these zones, similar for all four fingers, may appear theoretical, but there is a close association between the anatomical site and the clinical features. Study of the alteration in prehension in an amputee indicates what the most useful amputation level may be.

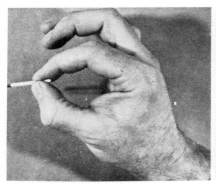
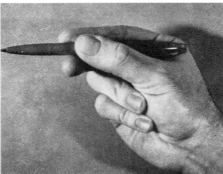
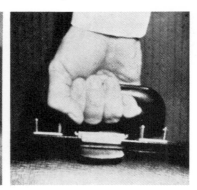

Figure 6.1
Digital pinch grip.

Figure 6.2
Digital pinch grip.

Figure 6.3
Palmar grip.

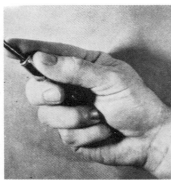
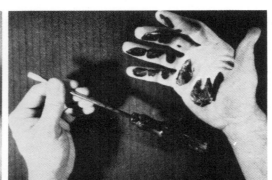

A   B

Figure 6.4
A and B, Directional grip showing finger prints including those of the palmar grip.

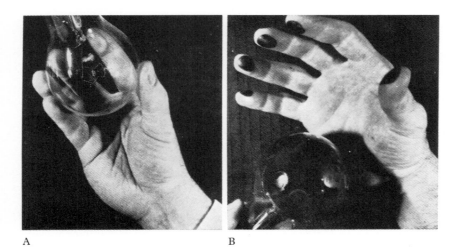

A   B

Figure 6.5
A and B, Multiple pulp grip (spherical grip) with finger prints on pulps.

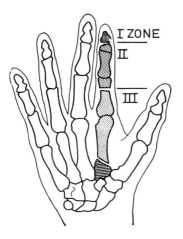

Figure 6.6
Definition of the three amputation levels as applied to the index finger.

AMPUTATION OF THE INDEX FINGER (FIG. 6.6)

Amputations of the index finger modify that digit which, after the thumb, is the most useful. It is essential for the pinch grip and also provides a stabilising factor in the palmar grip. Every amputation, however minimal the loss, alters prehension. As we have already said, there are, for each digit, amputation levels where problems are similar.

Zone I. This extends from pulp tip to base of distal phalanx and the aim is to preserve a satisfactory pulp in this zone. The functional importance of the pulp is well recognised and any reduction of this shortens the index finger in relation to the other pulps, altering the pinch grip.

The patients either do not use or use only awkwardly, the thumb/index pinch for picking up small objects (Moberg's picking-up test between one and six out of ten). The thumb/index pinch might only be ued as a pre-tip radial opposition, the middle finger tending to replace the index for tip-to-tip pinch (Fig. 6.7). Lastly, the directional grip and the multiple (spherical) grip are altered to a less extent and there is no change in the palmar grip.

In studying the functional alterations of the four grips one may apportion a score for each, ranging from one to four.

From the practical point of view, it is quite apparent that maximum length should be preserved and a satisfactory pulp provided in this zone. This zone may be divided into two parts:

1. Amputations of the distal third, obliquely or transversely in such a way as to leave a pulp after amputation.

All the available reconstructive techniques have been used, depending on the circumstances, to preserve maximum length (direct suture, free grafts, local flaps). We do not intend describing them since they have been studied in detail by Gosset's report (Gosset and Michon, 1965).

Unless suture, which is the ideal is possible, we use skin grafts. We do not use flaps from elsewhere as we feel they interfere with a normal area without having a major advantage.

Lastly, preservation of the nail root allows regrowth of the nail.

2. Amputations of the distal 2/3. These cases present different problems. The nail cannot be preserved so the nail root should be excised. The remaining pulp of the stump will not be adequate to provide a useful new pulp. The methods of providing skin cover already detailed for distal 1/3 injuries are also used for this region. The problems raised by amputation through the base of the distal phalanx will be discussed in the section devoted to problems seen in zone II.

Removal of the base of the distal phalanx does not affect movement of the remaining stump because each phalanx has its own tendon attachments but the power of the pinch grip is considerably diminished by loss of flexor digitorum profundus and the extensor tendon. This means, therefore, that the base of the distal phalanx should be saved whenever possible.

Zone II (Fig. 6.8). This lies between the base of the distal phalanx and the head of the proximal phalanx. Here the aim is to save a mobile useful index stump.

The lack of pulp and nail is the main concern. The middle finger takes over from the index for digital pinch and patients find writing difficult. The palmar grip is altered owing to lack of the winding-up action of the index finger. The multiple pulp grip is also affected but the residual index finger stump is still useful in assisting the directional grip.

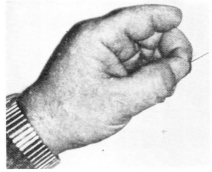
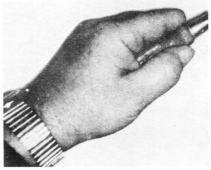

Figure 6.7
Amputation of the index finger in zone I. The middle finger tends to replace the index for tip-to-tip pinch.

D

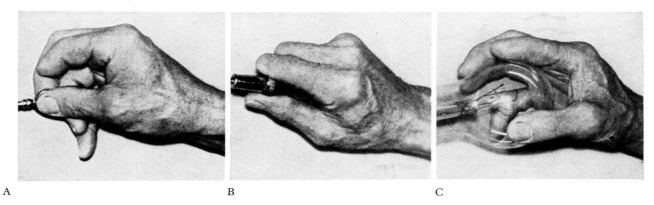

A   B   C

Figure 6.8
A, B and C, Amputation of the index finger in zone II. Middle finger replaces index for pinch grip. Stump still useful for directional grip but spherical grip reduced.

Any amputation stump in zone II is useful and should be preserved by simple surgical means even if this involves shortening the bone 1 to 2 millimetres. Mobility of the remaining joints (P.I.P. and M.P.) is essential.

Zone III (Fig. 6.9A, B, C). Between head of proximal phalanx and base of the metacarpal.

It is here that we are concerned more than at any other site with the optimal level of an elective amputation. There are always the alternatives of either preserving a short index stump, base of proximal phalanx or head of metacarpal, or amputating through the metacarpal base.

The arguments in favour of retaining a stump are that one preserves maximum width of the hand and support for a tool handle without appreciably reducing the power of the hand in a manual worker.

These are valid arguments but we feel that amputation at the base of the 2nd metacarpal discussed by Gosset (Gosset and Michon, 1965) and Chase (1968) is preferable. Indeed,

such an amputation provides a maximal spread of the thumb web and the middle finger takes on the function of the index and is more useful (Fig. 6.9).

Transfer of the 1st dorsal interosseus to the 2nd dorsal interosseus muscle enables this finger to be deviated to the radial side in making a most effective pinch between it and the thumb (Fig. 6.10).

Manual dexterity is better than when a stump is left since this is likely to be awkward and useless. The hand also has a better cosmetic appearance.

AMPUTATION OF MIDDLE FINGER (FIG. 6.11)

Amputation of the middle finger changes the function of the longest finger which normally supports the index in the pinch grip and fills the gap between index and ring fingers preventing small objects falling out of the palm.

Zone I. Difficulties encountered in the various grips are appreciable except the multiple finger grip in which the

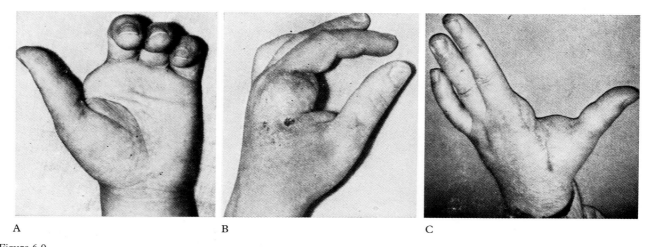

A   B   C

Figure 6.9
A, B, and C, Amputation of index finger in zone III near the metacarpal base. This results in maximal spread of thumb web with the middle finger taking over the function of the index.

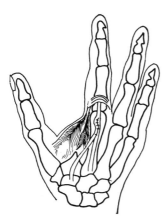

Figure 6.10
Transfer of first dorsal interosseous to second.

middle finger amputated at this level is not needed. This seems to us an important point.

Zone II. The pinch is good but the patient has difficulty in writing and the grip is reduced. Maximum length must be preserved to prevent overlapping of the fingers, small objects from falling out of the hand and to provide support (ulnar) for the index.

Zone III. Here again there is the problem of the optimal level for an elective amputation. The problems are important because a gap will remain between the fingers and allow small objects to fall out when the hand is closed. The index finger, being the first one and the other fingers incline towards one another (Fig. 6.12). This deviation of the fingers results in loss of prehensile strength since the line of pull of the tendons too, is also shifted. The pinch grip is weakened due to lack of support on the ulnar side and writing is difficult. Ablation of the 3rd metacarpal causes an even greater disability and we do not feel, like Caroll (1959), that this will overcome problems encountered with an injury through the base of the proximal

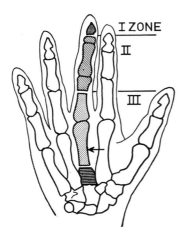

Figure 6.11
Amputation levels in middle finger.

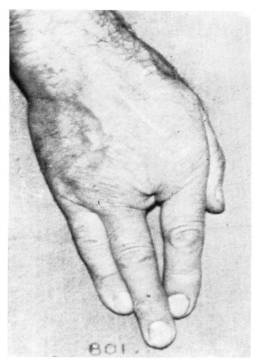

Figure 6.12
Amputation of middle finger in zone III.

phalanx or the metacarpal head. In fact, the 2nd metacarpal is fixed and the 4th slightly mobile so that the intermetacarpal space will remain open.

We feel in all amputations between middle of proximal phalanx and metacarpal base, with the exception of those patients who are symptom free or who have resumed normal activity, transfer of the whole index ray using the technique described by many authors and recently reviewed by Razemon (1969) will prevent the disabilities already described. The deep transverse intermetacarpal ligament should be reconstructed. The results following such a transfer are satisfactory from both functional and cosmetic points of view (Fig. 6.13A, B and C). Admittedly, the power is reduced because of the decrease in size of the hand but both the pinch grip and the multiple finger grip are improved.

AMPUTATION OF RING FINGER (FIG. 6.14)

Amputation of the ring finger alters that finger which, together with the little finger, complete the metacarpal arch. Because of the mobility of its metacarpal it participates in the mobile part of the metacarpal arch.

Zone I. Disability is minimal but the multiple finger grip is affected.

Zone II. Power of the palmar grip is reduced but disability is minimal if the stump is mobile; the finger does not wind-up. An amputation stump in this zone is useful in the same way as following similar amputation of the middle finger.

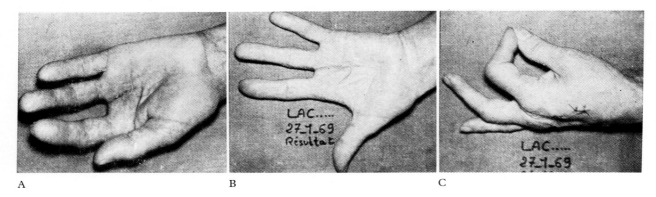

A   B   C

Figure 6.13
A, B and C, Index finger transfer for amputation of middle finger in zone III.

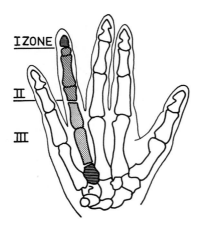

Figure 6.14
Amputation levels in ring finger.

Zone III. Deciding the optimal level for an elective amputation is difficult. Amputation through the middle or base of the
proximal phalanx presents a number of snags which we have
already encountered in the middle finger. These relate to
inclination of the fingers on flexion (Fig. 6.15), dropping out
of small objects from the closed hand and finally a loss of
power and weakness of the palmar grip.

The directional gripping function, on the contrary, is not
much affected (Fig. 6.16A and B). Transfer of the little finger
may improve function and appearance but there are a number
of inherent problems in this procedure which should be
mentioned, for example, reduction of the palm and ablation
of the 5th metacarpophalangeal joint both of which alter, to a
certain extent, the stabilising and securing role of the ring
finger. Besides, it seems to us, that contrary to the results of
amputation of the 3rd metacarpal, amputation of the 4th
metacarpal produces good results. In fact, the very mobile
5th metacarpal tends to close the 4th intermetacarpal space.
Amputation of the 4th metacarpal is performed by preserving
its base so as to maintain the joint relationship. The deep
transverse intermetacarpal ligament is reconstructed between
the 3rd and 5th metacarpals (Fig. 6.17).

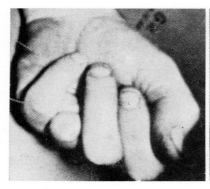

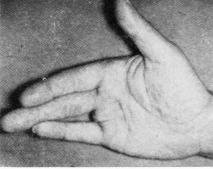

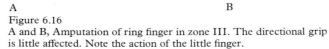

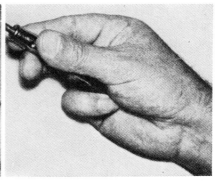

A   B

Figure 6.15   Figure 6.16
Amputation of ring finger in zone III.   A and B, Amputation of ring finger in zone III. The directional grip
                                            is little affected. Note the action of the little finger.

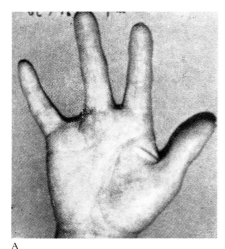

A

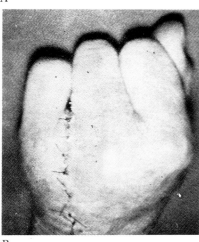

B

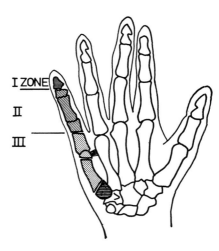

Figure 6.18
Amputation levels in little finger.

Figure 6.17
A and B, Mme LEV., 24.4.1970. Resection of 4th metacarpal for amputation of ring finger through the base of the proximal phalanx.

AMPUTATION OF LITTLE FINGER (FIG. 6.18)

Amputation of the little finger is of particular importance when one recalls that this finger is the key one on the ulnar side in controlling directional grip. If the gripping power is, above all, dependent on the strength of the middle and ring fingers which grasp the object in the palm, it is the little finger which prevents it from slipping. Mobility of the 5th carpometacarpal joint is essential. Lastly, the little finger plays a secondary part in controlling fine movements and prehension by extending the ulnar border of the palm (writing, drawing).

Zones I and II. Maximum length of the little finger must be preserved. The middle phalanx should be kept at all costs since movement at proximal interphalangeal and metacarpophalangeal joints is essential for directional grip.

Zone III. A stump in the region between the base of the proximal phalanx or even its head, and the metacarpophalangeal joint can no longer provide a blocking action on

this ulnar side and the directional grip is reduced (Fig. 6.19). It is, however, useful for prolonging the ulnar side of the hand. In certain cases, where the stump lacks mobility this may interfere with movements of the ring finger and should this be awkward it is better to amputate through the metacarpal.

Amputation through the metacarpophalangeal joint is troublesome and the appearance often ugly. It is better to amputate proximal to the head of the metacarpal but preserving the deep transverse intermetacarpal ligament to avoid abnormal mobility of the 5th metacarpal (Fig. 6.20).

Lastly, if amputation is to be undertaken through the shaft of the metacarpal, it is preferable to take it back to the base.

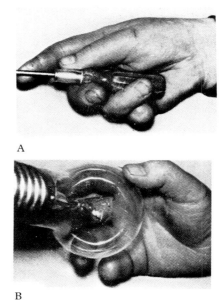

A

B

Figure 6.19
A and B, Amputation of little finger in zone III.

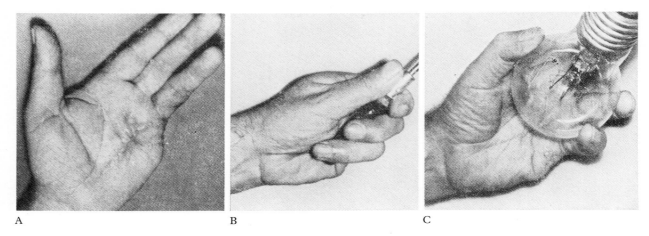

Figure 6.20
A, B and C, Amputation of little finger through metacarpal neck.

CONCLUSION

The optimal levels for amputation of any one finger which we have outlined in our series resulted from a study of the complications which may follow amputation. It is difficult to be precise about these levels and various factors have to be taken into account, for example, whether the involved finger is on the right or left hand, the age of the patient and the type of work he does. There are, however, at certain levels in each finger amputation sites where the problems are identical. These are particular points which may be settled at once but others can only be decided after studying the degree of functional adaptation. This particularly applies when considering transposition of fingers.

An understanding of these problems often enables one to improve on the inherent defects of all amputations.

Finally, both functional and cosmetic aspects have to be taken into account. Whilst certain operations undertaken primarily for a functional result also improve the cosmetic appearance, other operations cannot avoid the wearing of a prosthesis which may raise social problems.

BIBLIOGRAPHY

ALNOT, J.-Y. & ROUX, J. P. (1971). Possibilitiés et indications des traitements chirurgicaux dans les mutilations partielles de la main et des doigts. *Revue du praticien (Paris)*, **21**, 507–523.
CAROLL, R. E. (1959). Transposition of the index finger to replace the middle finger. *Clinical Orthopaedics*, **15**, 27.
CAROLL, R. E. (1959). Levels of amputation in the third finger. *American Journal of Surgery*, **97**, 477.
CHASE, A. (1968). The damaged index digit. A source of components to restore the crippled hand. *Journal of Bone and Joint Surgery*, **50A**, 1152.
CLAYTON, M. L. (1963). Index ray amputation. *Surgical Clinics of North America*, **43**, 367.
CRENSHAW, A. H. (1963). *Traité de chirurgie orthopédique de la clinique Campbell* Tome I, 4th Edition. Lee Milford.
DUPARC, J., ALNOT, J.-Y. & MAY, P. (1970). Amputations typiques de doigts. *Annales de chirurgie*, **24**, C. 1369–1377.
GOSSET, J. & MICHON, J. (1965). *67th Congrès de Chirurgie*, Paris.
ISELIN, M. (1967). *Traité de chirurgie de la main*. Paris, Ed. Méd. Flammarion.
KAPLAN, E. B. (1958). Replacement of an amputated middle metacarpal and finger by transposition of the index finger. *Bulletin of the Hospital for Joint Diseases, (N.Y.)*, **27**, 103.
LITTLER, J. W. (1960). Les principes architecturaux et fonctionnels de la main. *Revue de chirurgie orthopédique et réparatrice de l'appareil moteur*, **46**, 131.
PULVERTAFT, R. G. (1966). Severe combined mutilations of the thumb and fingers. Paris: S.I.C.O.T.
RAZEMON, J. P. (1969). Les transpositions de doigts. *Communication à la réunion du groupe d'étude de la main*. Paris.
SLOCUM, D. B. & PRATT, D. R. (1946). The principles of amputations of the fingers and hand. *Journal of Bone and Joint Surgery*, **26**, 535.
SWANSON, A. B. (1964). Levels of amputation of fingers and hand. Consideration for treatment. *Surgical Clinics of North America*, **44**, 1115.
TUBIANA, R. (1965). Mutilations sévères bilaterales des mains. *Amer. Chir. plast.*, **10**, 123.
VILAIN, R. & MICHON, J. (1970). *Chirurgie plastique cutanée de la main*. Paris.

7. AMPUTATION OF THE INDEX FINGER BY THE CHASE METHOD

M. Jandeaux and R. Kanhouche

Amputation of the index finger close to its base with transfer of the 1st dorsal interosseous muscle to the middle finger is an elegant way of dealing with many mutilating injuries of the index finger. The level at which the bone is divided together with the muscle transfer puts this procedure into a category far beyond that of the unsatisfactory standard amputations. The 1st dorsal interosseous, it should be noted, is the most powerful of the intrinsic muscles.

If an amputated index finger is still to be of use when all or part of the middle phalanx has been retained, there is a critical level in the middle phalanx proximal to which it is inadvisable to go, otherwise an unsatisfactory stump will be left in the thumb web. In 1946, Mahoney, Phalen and Frackleton observed the beneficial effects of metacarpal amputation of the index in 18 of their patients. This technique was modified by Chase in 1960, its principle features being as follows:

Proximal amputation of the index finger leaving only the minimum length of metacarpal necessary to conserve the width of the metacarpal arch
Transfer to the middle finger of the 1st dorsal interosseous and eventually of the extensor of the index to increase the functional capacity of the middle finger. This allows the hand to maintain its maximum grip
Establishment of a large web between thumb and middle finger which enhances both pinch and grasp. These functions are often affected by an index finger stump which is too short.

OPERATIVE TECHNIQUE

1. The skin incision (Fig. 7.1) is a racket type made up of two components:

A circular one circumscribing the metacarpophalangeal joint
A dorsal one, straight or lazy S along the radial side of the extensor expansion of the index finger.

It is helpful to direct this incision slightly towards the thumb, keeping it parallel to the 2nd metacarpal so that the eventual scar will lie more on the radial side than on the dorsum and so be less visible. It is also advisable to prolong this latter part of the incision sufficiently proximal so as to be able to amputate the metacarpal at the level of choice. A 'Z' may be included in this incision so as to enlarge the web, should this be required in very special cases.

The initial resection of a diamond shaped area of dorsal skin, as advocated by Chase, seems to us seldom indicated because this leaves a dorsal scar. Excess skin can always be trimmed at the end of the operation.

2. The neurovascular bundles are exposed on the palmar aspect:

Both arteries are ligated
The two nerves are cut back as proximally as possible exerting slight traction. The proximity of the division of the common volar digital nerve during this procedure must be constantly borne in mind. It is essential, however, because, as will be seen, one of the principal complications of the Chase amputation is the appearance of painful neuromata resulting from inclusion of the nerve ends in the scar.

3. The flexor tendons are cut after exerting traction on them. The aim again is to section them at the most proximal level. This will avoid interfering with flexor tendon function in the other fingers should the cut tendon of the amputated finger become adherent to the scar (the profundus tendons to all four fingers are linked).

4. The metacarpal is then exposed after dividing the extensor tendons of the index finger. The periosteum is incised longitudinally and carefully raised in order to preserve as much of the interossei as possible. Furthermore, the 1st interosseous is thus isolated and detached from the index

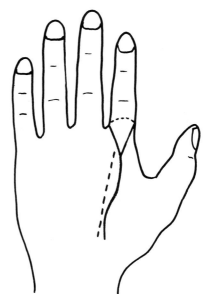

Figure 7.1
Skin incision.

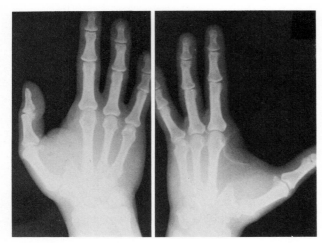

Figure 7.2
Level of amputation.

finger. The bone is divided about 1·5 cm from the carpo-metacarpal joint which exposes the insertion of the adductor pollicis.

As a rule, the bone is divided obliquely from below and towards the ulnar side but it would seem preferable to undertake this in a horizontal plane to avoid any protrusion into the new web (Figs. 7.2 and 7.3).

5. The detached insertion of the 1st dorsal interosseous is then fixed to the insertion of the 2nd interosseous at the level of the base of the proximal phalanx by two or three transfixion stitches of non-absorbable material. The 1st and 2nd dorsal interossei cover the site of bone section and provide padding over it.

The extensor digitorum of the index finger may be linked to that of the middle finger in such a way as to give to the latter independent extension, essential for pointing the finger. This junction must be adjusted in flexion to get the tension right. We do not perform it as a routine.

6. Skin closure is by interrupted sutures after placing a small suction drain in the wound. It is useful to place the scar towards the radial side, trimming palmar rather than dorsal skin if there is an excess of skin. A compression dressing is applied for 4 days. The fingers are mobilised at a very early stage.

One may take tension off the interosseous suture by means of a small wedge placed in the third web space holding the middle finger in slight abduction. In addition, the metacarpophalangeal joint is held in 30° of flexion.

ADVANTAGES OF THIS METHOD

What are the advantages of this simple procedure?

They may be classed as functional, cosmetic and psychological.

1. From a *functional* point of view, in fact, transfer of the 1st dorsal interosseous and the establishment of a large and supple thumb web provide the hand with a virtually normal range of usage. The presence of an index finger stump when the fingers are extended considerably interferes with function (Figs. 7.4, 7.5 and 7.6).

2. *Cosmetically* speaking the appearance of such a hand is satisfactory, the complete absence of the index finger not being unsightly or even apparent on casual observation.

3. This factor also explains the excellent results obtained from the *psychological* point of view. The patient is most likely to forget about his mutilating injury.

THE DISADVANTAGES

On the other hand, the drawbacks to the Chase operation are, in our opinion, minor ones.

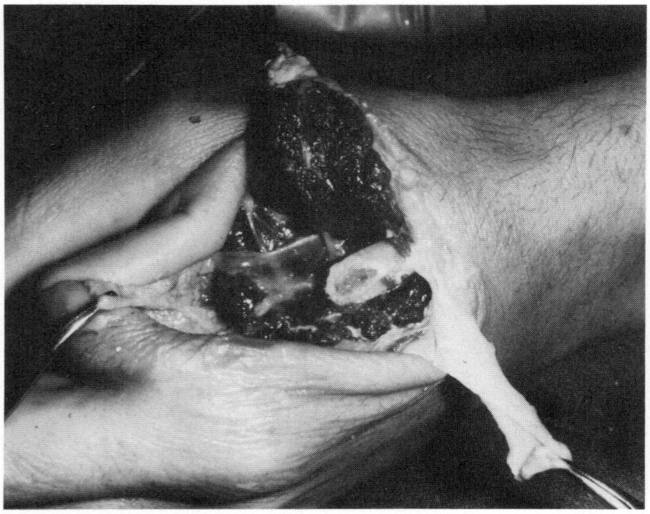

Figure 7.3
The metacarpal has been divided and the two motor units are isolated.

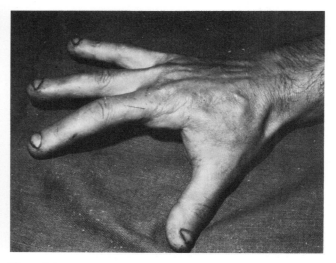

Figure 7.4
Result seen from the dorsal aspect.

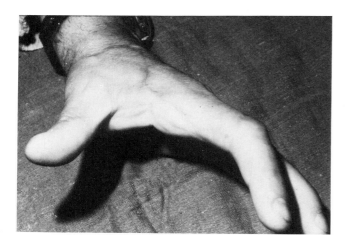

Figure 7.5
The resulting web.

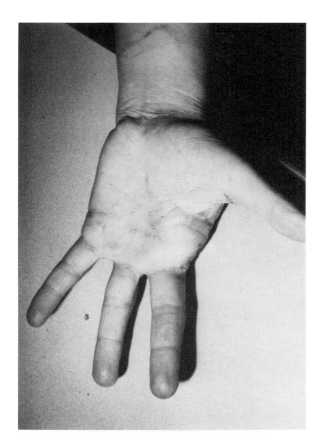

Figure 7.6
Result seen from the palmar aspect.

1. The spherical grasping force may be affected but early and intensive rehabilitation can minimise this deficiency. As a bonus, the middle finger receives the 'functional' heritage of the index finger due to the muscle and tendon transfer.

2. The prominence of the metacarpal stump on the dorsal aspect of the web has been noticeable. Division of the bone horizontally and the careful padding provided by the two interossei should rectify this fault.

Lastly, despite care taken in cutting back the digital nerves, neuromata are a not infrequent complication of this procedure.

THE INDICATIONS

Indications for the Chase amputation are numerous. This technique is indicated when stiffness, lack of sensation or even causalgia of the index finger seriously impair the function of the hand. It should be possible to know immediately when to proceed to metacarpal amputation, e.g. when the damage particularly to the neurovascular pedicles, rules out all hope of functional restoration.

However, this proximal, radical amputation will be envisaged only in the case of an isolated injury to the index finger. Where there are multiple amputations involving several fingers an index stump will be of use in secondary reconstruction. The various elements may be transferred to neighbouring sites (Chase).

Thus the dorsal skin may be used, for example, in constructing a flap for a contracted web. The remaining tendons and nerves may eventually be used as grafts. Lastly, the metacarpophalangeal stump will provide an excellent composite graft which, when transferred, will lengthen a thumb or shortened middle finger. In passing, it might be mentioned that this level of amputation is the optimal one when transferring an entire index finger either in a pollicisation or for replacement of an absent middle finger (Fig. 7.7).

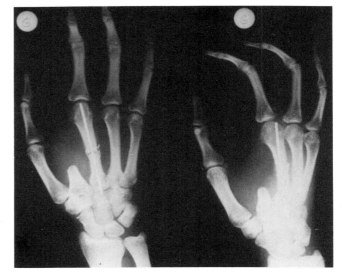

Figure 7.7
A digital transfer.

RESULTS

We have carried out this procedure on 35 occasions. We have not included in this series multiple mutilations in which the Chase technique has been used as a reconstructive measure (in the course of a digital transfer for example).

In these 35 cases, 10 late postoperative complications were relieved (nine neuromata and one case of stiffness of the middle finger).

Neuromata are relatively frequent. However, out of 29 manual workers 25 were able to return to their original work after a period of between 3 and 7 weeks. The spherical grasping force measured by a dynamometer appeared to be slightly reduced but was adequate in the majority of cases for sustained manual work.

This is a straightforward operation but it is more sophisticated and reconstructive in nature than the majority of standard amputations. The results, both cosmetic and functional, achieved by transferring to the middle finger the physiological characteristics of the index finger in this procedure should give it a place in the treatment of mutilating injuries of the hand.

BIBLIOGRAPHY

CHASE, R. A. (1960). Functional levels of amputation in the hand. *Surgical Clinics of North America*, **40**, 415–423.

CHASE, R. A. (1964). An attitude toward amputation in the hand. *Journal of the St Barnabas Medical Center*, **2**, 30–39.

CHASE, R. A. (1964). Conservation of usable structures in injured hands. *Reconstructive Plastic Surgery. Principle and Procedures in Correction. Reconstruction and Transplantation*, ed. Converse, J. M. Vol. 4, pp. 1579–1589. Philadelphia: W. B. Saunders.

CHASE, R. A. (1968). The damaged index digit. *Journal of Bone and Joint Surgery*, **50A**, 1152–1157.

DUNLOP, J. (1923). The use of the index finger for the thumb: some interesting points in hand surgery. *Journal of Bone and Joint Surgery*, **5**, 99–103.

GOTTLIEB, O. (1965). Metacarpal amputation: the problem of the four finger hand. *Acta chirurgica scandinavica*, **343**, suppl. 132–142.

LONDON, P. S. (1961). Simplicity of approach to treatment of the injured hand. *Journal of Bone and Joint Surgery*, **43B**, 454–464.

MAHONEY, J. H., PHALEN, G. S. & FRACKLETON, W. H. (1947). Amputation of the index ray. *Surgery*, **21**, 911–918

SLOCUM, D. B. & PRATT, D. R. (1944). The principles of amputations of the fingers and hand. *Journal of Bone and Joint Surgery*, **26**, 535–546.

VOLOIR, P. (1964). Niveaux d'amputation fontionnelle du pouce et des doigts. *Concours médical*, **86**, 5561–5571.

8. SURGICAL DIATHERMY IN THE PREVENTION AND TREATMENT OF AMPUTATION NEUROMATA OF THE FINGERS

J. Gosset

We are all aware of the serious functional disability which may result from these neuromata. We are continually seeing patients who, because of one of these neuromata, say they have been unable to return to work for months or even years.

The patient dreads the slightest contact with the stump which is painful. The physical disability progressively leads to disabling consequences. In the worst cases there is progressive causalgia, and personality disturbances are well recognised. We are not concerned here either with the clinical aspects or the causative mechanisms for which the neurologists, as yet, have no satisfactory explanation.

There is no denying the fact that treatment of painful amputation neuromata may be uncertain and confusing. We have all had cases where a simple digital neuroma has been treated by repeated amputations and a surgical 'ladder' leads to a sympathectomy and eventually even to a leucotomy. Prevention of amputation neuromata is therefore as important as their treatment is uncertain.

The majority of textbooks neglect this problem in those chapters devoted to amputations of the fingers. They deal with the elective sites for amputations. They discuss the design of the flaps and the techniques for closing unusual stumps where it is difficult to provide skin cover. Little is said of the essential management, which should be routine, of the divided ends of the digital nerves. One is generally advised to exert traction on the nerve and divide it as proximally as possible with or without application of a ligature. Frequently, however, both artery and nerve may be included in the same ligature. We consider this a mistake. We have no experience of ensheathing the nerve ends or of burying the nerve in a hole drilled in bone. This, in our view, complicates the procedure unnecessarily. We have met cases where failure after ensheathing the nerve end has been followed by further operations ending up with disastrous results.

The principle of our technique developed after a fortuitous finding. A male patient sustained a deep electric burn of the proximal part of the palm of the hand just distal to the wrist. The median nerve was destroyed over a length of several centimetres. At a further operation 3 months later, the proximal end of the damaged nerve seemed, to us, to have an unusual appearance. In actual fact, it ended in an almost pointed spindle with no evidence of a neuromatous swelling. We know that the cancer surgeons carrying out wide cervical gland clearances diathermise the superficial branches of the cervical plexus and that they say neuromata never occur in the scar.

For more than 15 years, we have routinely coagulated the nerve stumps with diathermy following amputation. We have tried to ensure that this same technique is also used by our assistants. It is virtually impossible to present the results statistically. We are in a position to state, however, that out of several hundred digital amputations only three patients, to our knowledge, operated on by young assistants, have produced neuromata necessitating secondary treatment. We cannot rule out the possibility, of course, that certain patients may have gone to other surgeons subsequently.

With these reservations, we remain convinced of the efficacy of surgical diathermy in the prevention of neuromata.

The technique is simple but requires care and precision. The operation is quick and does not require a pneumatic tourniquet. A simple elastic tourniquet applied at the wrist is always adequate.

It is never necessary to look for the end of the cut nerve at the site of its section or of the amputation. One must seek it more proximally at the base of the flap which will have been dissected from the bone, then raised and turned back by two lateral reflections. One finds the nerve in healthy tissue and always lying nearer the mid-line than one would have expected. The two digital nerves are then dissected throughout the length of the incision.

The end of the nerve is grasped very firmly by very fine forceps and drawn out so as to be free for at least a centimetre.

One then proceeds to the surgical diathermy. The diathermy electrode may be placed on any part of the body. The lead is attached to the forceps which hold the end of the nerve. Coagulation with the diathermy must only be with low intensity current. Excessive burning would slacken the forceps. One, therefore, begins with the lowest possible current and the theatre nurse may slowly increase its strength while the surgeon watches the appearance of the isolated nerve with the aid of a magnifying loupe. It is most important not to exert traction on the nerve but allow it to remain slack. Suddenly it begins to crumple, retract, sizzle, diminish in size and turn yellow. Maintaining this current one continues until these changes have occurred over a distance of 5 to 6 mm. Finally, one trims off with the scissors the terminal 2 to 3 mm of the nerve.

This procedure when used for amputations of the middle phalanx carries a certain risk when applying the diathermy at the level of the proximal phalanx. We noted this at the start of our trials. There is a risk of the nerve destruction reaching the division of the common volar digital nerve and then involving the nerve to the adjacent finger. Having had two such complications we modified the diathermy technique when used in the proximal parts of the finger. Here, diathermy must be bi-polar. One no longer uses an electrode, but the diathermy is applied between two forceps placed on the nerve 1 cm apart. The proximal forceps held by an assistant are connected by a crocodile tweezer to the lead which normally goes to the electrode. The diathermy apparatus is then attached by a lead to the distal forceps and the current is gently and progressively applied between the two forceps. The current is increased as gently as in the preceding cases and diathermy is stopped when the length of nerve between the two forceps is dried up, retracted and yellow.

The efficacy of this technique naturally led us to apply it to established amputation neuromata. There is obviously less chance of success when the neuroma is associated with pain up the limb and psychoneurotic complications. It is much more hopeful when the pain has a precise, limited site, localised to the neighbourhood of the scar. The diathermy technique is the same but the search for the neuroma sometimes presents difficulties. One approaches it at the level of the scar but it is important not to look for the neuroma in the scar tissue itself. One must raise an adequate flap to isolate the nerve in a scar-free area and at a distance from the scar. The flap must be thick and elevated from the bone. Having found the nerve trunk in healthy tissue one follows it from a proximal level distally. By this means one is led to the neuroma buried in fibrous tissue where it would otherwise be practically impossible to locate immediately. Even if, clinically, there is evidence of a single neuroma, it is preferable to diathermise both palmar digital nerves. In four cases we have found dorsal neuromata. Moreover, on two occasions the latter were recognised only at a subsequent operation which was crowned with success after a setback following diathermy applied only to palmar neuromata. Whenever the amputation scar is atrophic and closely applied to bone we undertake revision with trimming of bone in order to produce a better scar. Provided one adheres closely to the indications outlined above, and excluding those cases with pain up the limb, the success rate in these secondary operations is about 60 per cent.

9. THE PHALANGEAL HAND

R. Souquet and M. Mansat

The phalangeal hand may be defined as the mutilation resulting from the loss either simultaneously or successively, of several fingers but with preservation of the metacarpophalangeal joints.

This injury never seems to offer sufficient originality meriting a separate paper, when defined within these limits. The coexistence of several lesions does not alter the principles of plastic surgical repair, and principles which apply when a single finger is injured are all the more important in multiple lesions. However, it does seem that the presence of multiple lesions must modify one's general approach, make one more conservative regarding indications for ablation, and, above all, give us greater scope for reconstructive procedures. We feel that comparatively minor procedures are justified, e.g. slight lengthening of stumps, use of local flaps with sensation, localised deepening of certain webs, which would not even be considered in the case of a single lesion.

AETIOLOGY

Multiple digital injuries are the price paid for this modern industrial era. They are particularly common in certain jobs: carpenters injured by planes and especially by revolving machinery; printers crushed by presses; cleaners and workers with plastic material trapped by hot or cold presses.

For several years there have been two further factors which have tended to increase the incidence of these injuries: on the one hand, the swift mechanisation of agriculture in a population not yet accustomed to it, has increased these accidents, e.g. in stripping maize, crushing fodder etc.; on the other hand, the extraordinary spread of mechanical grass cutters has opened a new chapter of their type of injury in a social class which was previously not at risk.

Before presenting, step by step, the few thoughts we hope to pass on to you and although we are only concerned with the secondary repair, it is certainly useful to stress yet again the value of initial conservatism when faced with the problem of whether or not to perform a primary amputation. A single observation of ours seems to demonstrate this; it was the case of a young woman worker who was injured by a cardboard folding machine. Initially, there appeared to be severe damage to the index finger and a compound fracture with gross displacement of the middle finger which threatened serious ischaemia. In fact, on the fourth day, it was the ring finger which showed progressive gangrene necessitating amputation. Too hasty an ablation would only have made, what was a serious injury, even worse.

SECONDARY TREATMENT

We only intend discussing, in our paper, the management from a point of view of function. An intensive programme of surgical reconstruction solely for cosmetic reasons, does not seem to us to have any place whatever in treatment of the phalangeal hand, and in any case such a reconstruction falls far short of the perfection that a modern prosthesis provides.

However, it is quite obvious that there are some ugly stumps which require trimming. One in point is the disarticulation of the distal interphalangeal joint which is much improved by removal of its volar prominence and by trimming the condyles of the phalangeal head. This procedure can always be combined with the construction of a false nail bed by the method of González-Ulloa or a similar method.

MOBILISING PROCEDURES

Among the operations for improving function one must first discuss the mobilising procedures. Any means for increasing movement in a stump by mobilising a stiff joint is indicated. There is nothing so valuable as excision and grafting of contractures following palm burns which prevent satisfactory opening of the hand (Fig. 9.1). All the same, in complex

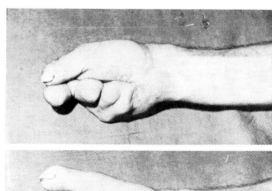
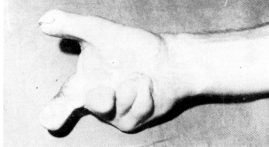

Figure 9.1
Loss of several phalanges due to a burn resulting in severe contracture necessitating excision and skin graft.

lesions where there is marked stiffness we feel that capsulectomies are indicated either of the metacarpophalangeal joints by the Bunnell method, or the interphalangeal joints where the collateral ligaments and the glenoid ligament are resected as described by Curtis.

The removal of flexor profundus or even both tendons in very proximal lesions may correct contractures due to excessive muscle tension or fibrous adhesions in the palm.

Our experience of joint prostheses, particularly those of Swanson, is too limited and too recent for us to discuss in detail but we do feel they are of considerable value in the management of stiff or ankylosed stumps which have sufficient length.

THE RE-ESTABLISHMENT OF SENSIBILITY

Multiple digital amputations are often associated with more or less complete loss of sensation due either to division of their nerves, or as a result of the stumps having been covered by a distant skin flap. Every effort must be made to cover the area which now acts as the pulp, with skin possessing as near normal innervation as possible. This is essential if the corresponding digital ray is to be used adequately.

Secondary suture of divided nerves is always indicated where possible even if this only leads to a return of protective sensibility.

The innervated skin pedicle is undoubtedly the ideal theoretical solution, but its practical realisation presents certain difficulties and at times is virtually impossible. The original technique of Littler, tempting in principle, elegant in its execution, efficient in its use, is rarely possible. The donor finger is often missing. When it is present, one hesitates to mutilate this intact element, at times the only one remaining.

It is necessary in most cases to resort to a different technique and one normally undertakes a local repair transferring a flap from the dorsal aspect.

The skin plasty using the same finger is simple and efficacious making use of the distal skin innervated by dorsal nerve branches. Such a flap may be used on a fresh defect or to replace a scarred area.

The metacarpal neck flap, incorporating the longitudinal nerve filaments, enables one, in very proximal amputations to provide cover of good quality, but also requires a further operation to re-fashion the web.

Raising a dorsal flap on an adjoining finger is often the only possible solution. The most elegant version is certainly the innervated skin flap, but in order to be practical and safe it is necessary to carry out a most detailed clinical investigation of the innervated area by blocking the different nerve trunks with local anaesthetic.

We wish to quote the following case which we consider unusual: this was a patient who had been crushed by an agricultural machine and presented with a major skin avulsion which had necessitated emergency treatment by an abdominal flap. The resulting disability, complicated by a stiff thumb from a previous injury, required surgical correction. In addition to freeing the index stump we covered its volar aspect with a large flap raised on the back of the thumb carefully preserving the minute nerve filaments. After a further operation involving excision and grafting on the palm of the hand the patient regained reasonable prehension and almost perfect sensibility of the stump (Fig. 9.2).

When there is partial loss of sensation on a stump due to division of one nerve, transferring the innervated zone into the centre of the pulp is of major importance. We will not touch on the problems of painful stumps, already dealt with in

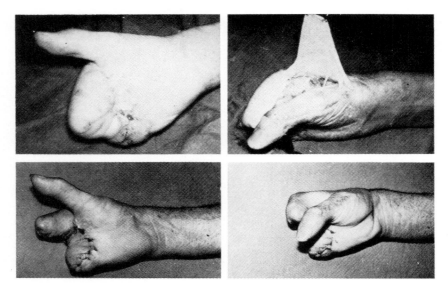

Figure 9.2
An innervated flap raised on the dorsum of the thumb, used to replace the abdominal flap, applied as primary skin cover to the index stump which was then phalangised.

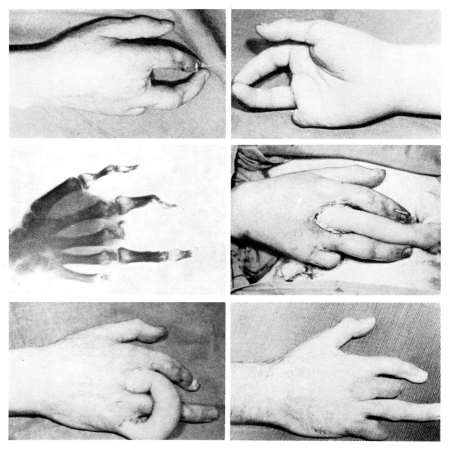

Figure 9.3
Tubed flaps with bone grafts to lengthen finger stumps which may improve appearance but which are usually useless from a functional point of view.

this symposium, other than to underline the importance of the subject.

LENGTHENING OPERATIONS

A lengthening procedure is nearly always unnecessary in a lesion limited to a single finger, and can only be justified in quite exceptional cases and for purely social reasons. On the contrary, in multiple finger injuries, a lengthening, even of minimal extent, may be very valuable. Ten to 15 mm of additional length can transform a useless stump into a functioning element necessary to complete or ensure the gripping of a tool. The essential factor which makes lengthening procedures useful is the preservation or re-establishment of adequate sensibility, be it only protective. This virtually excludes the use of distant flaps, of which we have had some experience, but which end in failure as in the case shown, where the attempted reconstruction of two amputated fingers gave a poor cosmetic result and a completely useless functional result (Fig. 9.3).

The most favourable case from the point of view of treat-

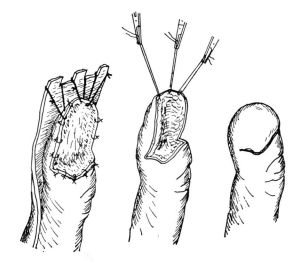

Figure 9.4
Technique for lengthening in the case of a typical amputation stump using a palmar flap.

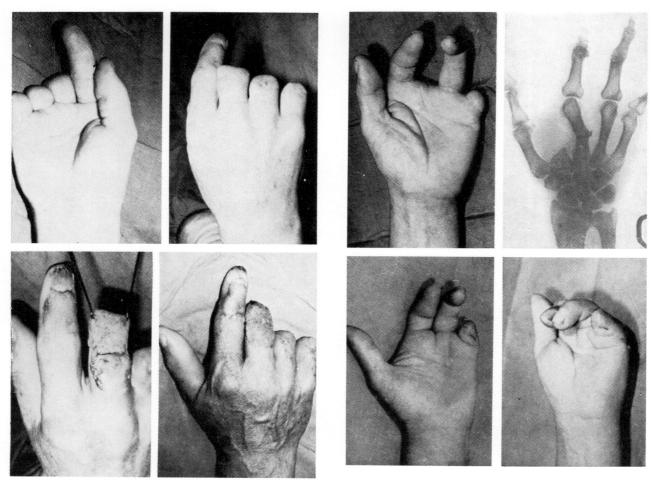

Figure 9.5
Application of this technique in a middle finger stump.

Figure 9.6
Arthrodesis of the proximal interphalangeal joints. Transfer of index finger to 3rd metacarpal; lengthening of little finger stump.

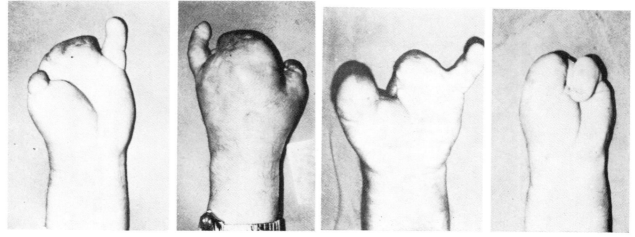

Figure 9.7
Transfer of metacarpophalangeal joint of index finger to 1st metacarpal.

ment is where, at the primary amputation, the ablation has left a large palmar flap which is extremely vascular and well innervated. It is then an easy matter to re-create the initial defect by re-opening the dorsal scar and releasing the flap. The secondary defect is then covered with a free graft or, if necessary, by a thoracic or forearm flap as the case may be. When the bone graft is not inserted at this stage, it is often useful, in order to prevent shrinkage of the flap, to fix its edges to a stent mould of adequate size (Figs. 9.4 and 9.5).

The same technique is eminently suitable in oblique amputation on either side which must then be repaired by a distant flap. As a secondary procedure it is necessary to centralise the skin with intact sensation. In a number of cases, reconstruction of the initial flap is either impossible or does not apply. One must then resort to a dorsal flap of the flag type but a combination of this with a stump lengthening is always a most hazardous procedure.

The techniques of lengthening which we have suggested are only, as a rule, part of a more major reconstruction in a mutilated hand involving various procedures which other authors have already discussed, e.g. transfer of digits, ampu-tation of useless or troublesome elements, web adjustment. We only wish to quote two cases in concluding this paper.

The first one, a joiner, sustained amputation of middle and little fingers complicated by ankylosis of the interphalangeal joints in bad positions. The particular problem here was to replace these joints in a functional position, i.e. of semiflexion and to balance the palm by transferring the second digital ray on to the third metacarpal, and finally to produce a minimal but effective lengthening of the stump of the base of the proximal phalanx of the little finger (Fig. 9.6).

The second patient, also a woodworker, presented, in addition to thumb loss through the metacarpal, loss of the middle three digits and had been treated by a primary abdominal flap. Reconstruction consisted of transfer of the metacarpophalangeal joint of the index finger to the 1st metacarpal with deepening of the 1st web whilst carefully preserving the neurovascular skin connections.

The result shows, as well as a satisfactory prehensile pinch that the tactile surfaces are covered with skin of normal sensibility which is equally good for the power grip as for picking up small objects (Fig. 9.7).

E

10. PHALANGISATION OF THE METACARPALS

R. Tubiana

Deepening the webs, when 'phalangising' the metacarpals, improves the intermetacarpal pinch. This procedure is particularly useful with the peripheral metacarpals which are the only mobile ones.

The 2nd and 3rd metacarpals are fixed, articulating with the distal row of carpal bones. These carpometacarpal joints have virtually no movement. Together they form the stable element of the metacarpal arch. The peripherally placed metacarpals on the other hand possess variable degrees of mobility: this is quite considerable for the 1st metacarpal which can oppose against the other metacarpals, and much less, though extremely useful, for the 5th metacarpal which as it goes to meet the opposing 1st metacarpal can flex 20° to 35° anterior to the plane of the fixed metacarpals.

The 4th metacarpal possesses even more restricted mobility: some 10° of flexion which contributes to cupping of the hand. This is too small a range to be used for independent grasp.

Phalangisation is performed mostly in cases of severe mutilation of the hand with the loss of several fingers. It may also be beneficial in severe stiffness, when contracture of the soft tissues prevents normal movement of the mobile metacarpals.

We shall consider in turn phalangisation of the 1st metacarpal, of the 5th metacarpal, and finally the combined phalangisation of both 1st and 5th metacarpals.

PHALANGISATION OF THE 1ST METACARPAL

Phalangisation of the 1st metacarpal consists in deepening the 1st web. It was performed by Huguier as early as 1873.

ANATOMICAL CONSIDERATIONS

The 1st intermetacarpal space is in fact a hinge, with extreme mobility, which makes opposition of the thumb possible. For normal abduction, anteposition, adduction and rotation to occur, the soft tissues, especially on the dorsal aspect, must be extremely supple. Any scar or skin contracture will reduce the range of movements of the 1st metacarpal. Every phalangisation, therefore, must provide ample skin covering.

The intermetacarpal space is filled by two muscles which are triangular in shape and cross over each other. Anteriorly lies adductor pollicis which arises mainly from the 3rd metacarpal; it has a tendinous insertion on the medial sesamoid of the thumb as well as dorsal phalangeal expansions. Its transverse fibres form the 'bow-string' of the web. Lying more posteriorly is the 1st dorsal interosseous which is attached to the medial border of the 1st metacarpal and has

a tendinous insertion to the base of the proximal phalanx of the index finger.

Any significant deepening of the 1st web will require detachment of these two muscles to a greater or lesser degree.

The muscles are covered on their superficial aspects by two aponeuroses, one palmar and one dorsal. An apponeurotic sheet passes from each of these to line the deep surfaces of the muscles. These fibrous structures are all liable to contract following an injury which requires immobilisation. They must therefore be incised plane by plane. The dorsal capsule of the trapezometacarpal joint, which is normally very lax, may also contract, in which case it will have to be incised.

OPERATIVE TECHNIQUE

The incision must give a good exposure of the structures in both anterior and posterior aspects of the web; one must also be prepared to add skin, either as a flap or a free graft. We

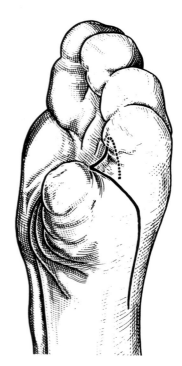

Figure 10.1
Incisions outlined for phalangisation of 1st metacarpal: a Z-plasty is used in the web; the palmar incision is extended on to the thenar eminence; the dorsal incision extends to the carpometacarpal joint of the thumb or even to the wrist to free the extensor tendons if necessary.

usually start with a Z-type incision straddling the web; the anterior limb follows the opposition crease; the posterior limb must be such that it can be extended proximally to the trapezometacarpal joint, or even further should it become necessary to free the dorsal extrinsic tendons of the thumb on the back of the wrist (Fig. 10.1).

Anteriorly, the two neurovascular bundles of the thumb and the radial neurovascular bundle of the index finger are carefully dissected out; posteriorly, the sensory branches of the radial nerve are also isolated and mobilised. The anterior and posterior aponeuroses are incised from end to end; the deep fibrous sheet and all the tight fibrous structures stretched between the 1st two metacarpals are incised in turn.

The muscles are dealt with according to the circumstances. The 1st dorsal interosseus is only worth saving when there is an index stump present. It is usually only partially detached from the 1st metacarpal, its attachment to the second metacarpal being left intact. If required, its action as an abductor of the index finger may be restored by transferring the extensor indicis proprius. Adductor pollicis, however, is much more difficult to deal with when one is attempting to deepen the web, and its function must be restored after a phalangisation. In cases where it has retained its contractility, it must be spared as far as possible.

If only a limited degree of deepening is required, as in partial amputation of the thumb, it is adequate to use the technique for preventing contracture, i.e. detaching the distal fibres from the 3rd metacarpal. When more extensive deepening is indicated, however, it will be necessary to detach the sesamoid tendon of the adductor and re-implant it halfway down the shaft of the 1st metacarpal (Fig. 10.2). If the muscle is markedly fibrotic, it is preferable to free most of its attachment and to reinforce its action by means of a powerful tendon transfer. We ourselves have used flexor pollicis longus or the flexor of an amputated finger for that purpose. The transferred tendon is implanted into the 1st metacarpal and passed through a small tunnel in the bone. When the whole muscle is fibrotic one may have to excise it before doing the transfer.

We have mentioned earlier that the movements of the 1st metacarpal may be hampered by tendinous adhesions on the posterior aspect of the wrist. We have seen such cases following crush injuries of the forearm, leading to ischaemic changes and sometimes mutilation of the extremities. It is important to make sure that the trapezometacarpal joint has maintained sufficient mobility; if the movements are still limited after a dorsal capsulectomy, an arthroplasty must be considered. Instead of the simple excision of the trapezium which was once employed, we now prefer to replace the bone by a silastic implant.

The skin covering can be dealt with in one of several ways, depending on the degree of deepening achieved and on the state of the adjacent soft tissues. If minimal phalangisation is required, a Z-plasty may be sufficient. In the presence of a healthy graft bed, a full-thickness graft may often have to be used in addition. Otherwise, a skin flap will be necessary. This can be taken from an adjacent area on the dorsal aspect of the

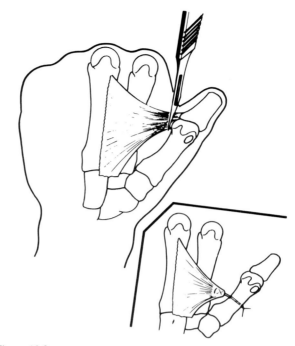

Figure 10.2
Dividing the adductor insertion which is re-attached more proximally on the 1st metacarpal allowing deepening of the web.

hand if the soft tissue is supple, or preferably from the opposite limb, especially if there is a wide area to be covered. The flap must be thin and stripped of its fatty layer to avoid filling up the newly constructed commissure. Ideally, pressure areas should be covered with sensitive skin.

PHALANGISATION OF THE 5TH METACARPAL

We described the technique for this operation in 1958 but subsequently modified it appreciably (Tubiana and Roux, 1974).

The incision is made in relation to the 4th metacarpal but more on the dorsal than the palmar aspect of the hand, in order to preserve skin with sensibility on the lateral aspect of the 5th metacarpal, or at least at the extremity of the stump. The incision should be S-shaped or angled to prevent risk of contracture. The dorsal longitudinal veins should be preserved as far as possible. Anteriorly, the digital artery and the nerve of the 4th interspace are traced down to their division. The digital artery to the ulnar site of the ring finger is tied and divided. The nerve is freed to the proximal part of the palm. The transverse intermetacarpal ligament is then divided.

All hypothenar muscles with their carpal origins are preserved. It is the deepest, the opponens digiti minimi, which alone is directly attached to the 5th metacarpal and which exerts the most marked action on the movements of that bone. The abductor brevis and flexor brevis of the little finger are inserted on the ulnar side of the base of the proximal phalanx and only have an indirect action. The 3rd palmar interosseus,

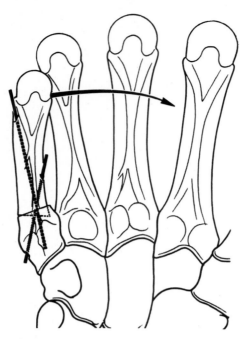

Figure 10.3
Phalangisation of the 5th metacarpal. Osteotomy near the base of the 5th metacarpal and angulation of the distal part forward and radially.

which arises from the 5th metacarpal and inserts into the radial side of the base of the proximal phalanx of the little finger, is transferred to the ulnar side and thus acquires a pronating action. The 4th dorsal interosseus, which is inserted on the base of the proximal phalanx of the ring finger, is removed. An osteotomy is performed at the base of the 5th metacarpal through a dorsal incision. The bone is divided with an oscillating saw about 1·5 cm from the carpometacarpal joint. The intermetacarpal space is split proximally as far as the deep palmar arch and the deep branch of the ulnar nerve which is carefully preserved. The distal part of the metacarpal is angled forward and radially (Fig. 10.3). The position at the osteotomy site is held by two Kirschner wires which, obviously, must not interfere with the movements of the adjacent joint. A posterior capsulectomy of the metacarpohamate joint may be performed with division of the oblique posteromedial ligament, the stabilising proximal intermetacarpal ligament of the joint being preserved. Finally, a full-thickness skin graft, from the forearm, is used to cover the web.

INDICATIONS FOR PHALANGISATION

Phalangisation of the 1st metacarpal only is indicated in cases of partial amputation of the thumb as well as in cases of simultaneous mutilation of the thumb and of the fingers.

1. In mutilation of the thumb at the proximal phalanx, a major reconstructive procedure of the thumb, such as pollicisation or reconstruction by tube pedicle, bone graft and island flap, seems hardly justified. A satisfactory alternative is to deepen the web to facilitate grasping of larger objects. This can be combined with lengthening of the thumb, by one centimetre or so using a bone graft covered by a local flap with sensibility.

2. Phalangisation of the 1st metacarpal is particularly useful when there is mutilation of both the thumb and the neighbouring fingers. It allows a pinch between the 1st and 2nd metacarpals. Lengthening the 1st metacarpal by any procedure is only of any value provided:

    a. there is sensation over the end of the stump.

    b. there are still finger-stumps against which the newly constructed thumb can oppose.

When there is a contracture of the thumb web and the index has been amputated, it is preferable to excise the 2nd metacarpal, preserving only its base to which the extensor carpi radialis is inserted, so as to ensure a wider grasp.

Phalangisation of the 5th metacarpal only is indicated when the four fingers have been amputated. If thumb function is present, pinching remains possible even though the four fingers have been lost. The shorter and the stiffer the thumb the more important is it to undertake phalangisation of the 5th metacarpal. Removal of the 4th metacarpal will widen the newly created commissure. This procedure which narrows the palm becomes unnecessary when the thumb is sufficiently

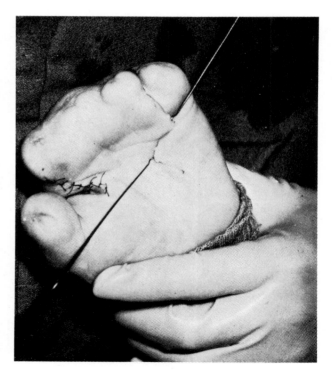

Figure 10.4
Phalangisation of 1st and 5th metacarpals. Incisions.

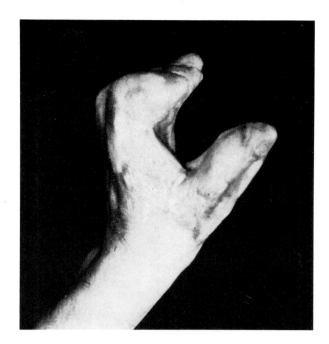

Figure 10.5
Phalangisation of 1st and 5th metacarpals. Result seen from radial side showing the span of the new thumb web.

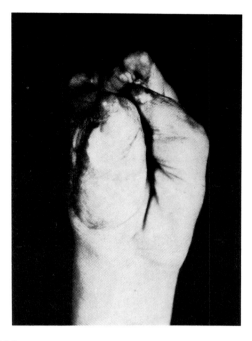

Figue 10.6
Phalangisation of the 1st and 5th metacarpals showing opposition between the 1st and 5th rays.

long to reach across and oppose the tip of the 5th metacarpal. It is useful, however, when thumb movements are limited or when the 5th metacarpal has been shortened. Part of the resected 4th metacarpal is used as a bone graft to lengthen the 5th metacarpal, and the lengthened bone is covered with a local skin flap carrying sensation.

Simultaneous phalangisation of the 1st and 5th metacarpals is indicated when the thumb and all four fingers have all been lost. It may provide a fair degree of useful prehension (Figs. 10.4, 10.5 and 10.6).

The essential element of the pinch is obviously the mobile 1st metacarpal. If the latter is stiff or has been lost, phalangisation of the 5th will achieve no useful purpose. In cases of amputation of the distal half, resection of the 2nd and 4th metacarpals will deepen the web. The 3rd metacarpal is kept in order to preserve the insertions of adductor pollicis; besides, the presence of this opposition post gives more precision to

the pinch when large objects are grasped. Very small objects (pins, sheets of paper) can be pinched between the 1st and 5th phalangised metacarpals.

With such phalangisations, sometimes performed on both hands, we have been able to restore independence to patients who had suffered severe bilateral mutilations.

BIBLIOGRAPHY

HUGUIER, P. C. (1973). Considérations anatomiques et physiologiques sur le rôle du pouce et sur la chirurgie de cet organe. *Archives générales de médecine*, **22**, 404, 567, 692, and (1974) **23**, 54.

TUBIANA, R. (1958). Phalangisation du 5me métacarpien. *Acta orthopaedica Belgica*, suppl. 3, 120.

TUBIANA, R. (1969). Repair of bilateral hand mutilations. *Plastic and Reconstructive Surgery*, **44**, 323.

TUBIANA, R. & ROUX, J. P. (1974). Phalangisation of the 1st and 5th metacarpals. *Journal of Bone and Joint Surgery*, **56A**, 447.

11. THE METACARPAL HAND

J. Michon

Amputation of the hand at metacarpal level may result from severe injury but a similar defect may be seen following failure of development in the congenital hand.

The problems of reconstruction vary greatly depending on the length of surviving metacarpal.

SHORT METACARPALS

The only solution in this situation, we maintain, consists in opposing the thumb metacarpal, provided it is of full length, to the stump of the hand built up by an iliac bone graft embedded in the 4th metacarpal. This block is then covered by a flap from elsewhere, generally the abdomen (Fig. 11.1).

This technique only restores a simple, basic grip between two surfaces but the two prehensile surfaces possessing sensibility enable a hand totally deprived of all prehension to regain some useful function. By this means, for example, a boy of 16 has been able to carry on the trade of arc welding. He can hold the welding torch with precision.

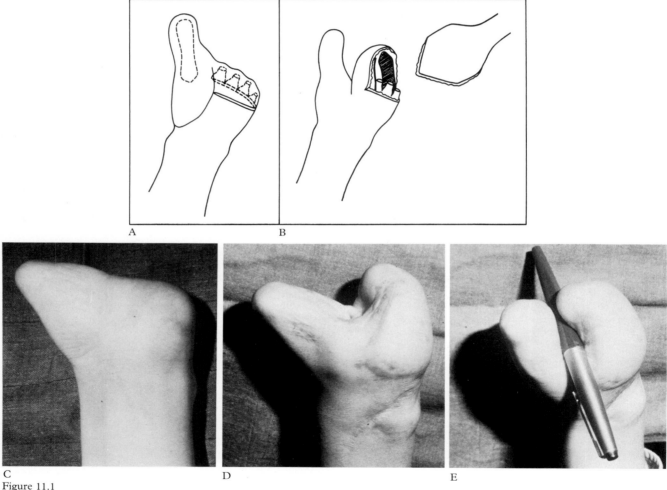

A   B

C   D   E

Figure 11.1
Raising of the palm as a flap; techniques for reconstruction of a prehensile pinch when the metacarpals are short.
A and B, The incision encircling the stump of which the soft tissues are raised whilst conserving the nerves. An iliac bone graft, carefully sited and secured supports the flap. The secondary defect is covered by an abdominal flap.
C, D and E, Case shown before and after reconstruction.

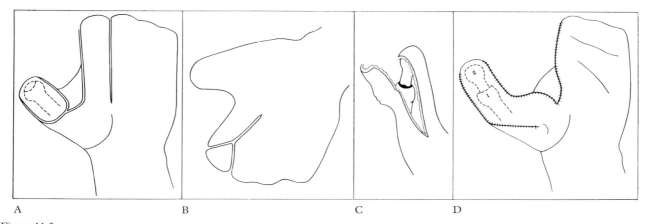

Figure 11.2
Pedicle transfer of the 2nd metacarpal to lengthen the thumb.
A, The incisions as seen from the palmar aspect.
B, The incisions from the dorsal aspect.
C, Lengthening of the thumb, the dorsal surface of which is here covered by raising the soft tissues of the palmar aspect.
D, Palmar aspect after skin suture.

LONG METACARPALS

There is much greater scope in these cases. Phalangisation of a metacarpal is a standard procedure, particularly where the 1st and 5th are concerned. Iselin (1961, 1967) long since published his technique for making a tripod hand and Tubiana (1958) added to it an osteotomy to angulate the 5th metacarpal which further improved function.

For our part, we consider that the best method for phalangisation of the 1st metacarpal is to remove the second ray which creates a large deep web necessary for grasping large objects.

There is a temptation to use this amputated metacarpal. Our experience has proved that it makes a poor free bone graft. Latterly, in order to lengthen the thumb, we have used a composite graft made up of a palmar skin strip from the index with its blood supply and innervation supplied by the neurovascular bundles together with the 2nd metacarpal, as for a digital transfer. Bony union is achieved by fixing the parts with pins or small plate and the residual raw areas following skin suture are covered as a rule by free grafts or occasionally by flaps should bare bone be exposed. These secondary defects, being on the dorsum or the side, sensation is not of cardinal importance.

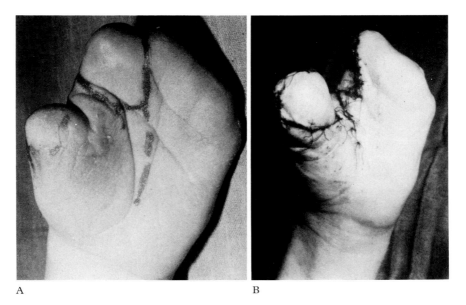

A   B

Figure 11.3
An example of the result of the technique shown in Fig. 11.2.

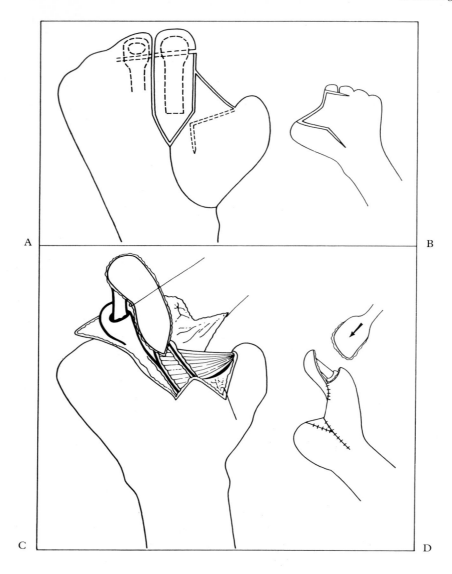

Figure 11.4
Pedicle transfer of the 2nd metacarpal to lengthen the 3rd ray.
A, Diagram of palmar incisions.
B, Dorsal incisions.
C, The oblique attachment of the transplanted segment on to the 3rd metacarpal head. The two neurovascular bundles of the index ensure its vascularity and innervation.
D, The reconstruction is completed by the dorsal skin cover. A flap is used here but frequently a free graft suffices.

In a certain type of mutilation which we have called 'thumb without finger', the thumb remains intact or only slightly shortened with the rest of the hand reduced to its metacarpals. Injuries with circular saws often cause this.

A similar type of reconstruction may be used in lengthening the 3rd metacarpal by transfer of the second ray. An increase in length here is made possible by extensive dissection of the pedicles making an island of the flap and attaching the 2nd metacarpal to the 3rd in 40 degrees of flexion.

The improved function brought about by these recon-structions has been appreciable in all cases, particularly for grasping large objects but also for the pinch, with the obvious limitations that the reconstructed extremity has, compared with the normal digital pulps when undertaking precision tasks.

We envisage, in fact, that a further step could be made in the treatment of the complete metacarpal hand. In addition to transferring the 2nd metacarpal to the 1st, one could also transfer the 4th to the 3rd or to the 5th. To date, our patients, satisfied with the result of the first procedure, have preferred

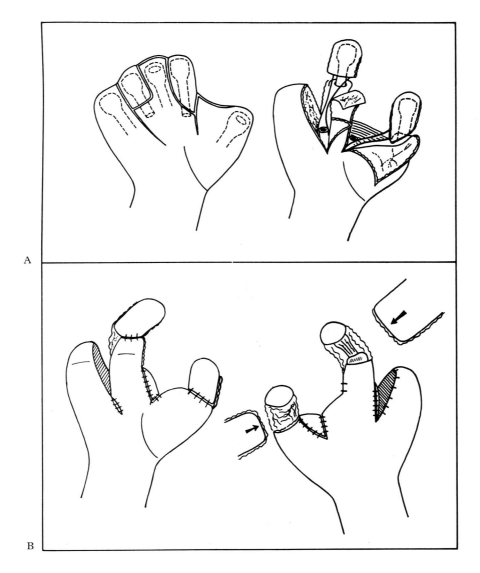

Figure 11.5
Double transfer: 2nd metacarpal on to 1st and 4th on to 3rd. It is advisable to carry out these two procedures at an interval of 2 to 3 months.
A, *Left:* the incisions on the palmar aspect. *Right:* transfer and attachment of the metacarpals showing the neurovascular bundles and skin flaps.
B, *Left:* palmar aspect after the transfer. *Right:* dorsal view. The secondary defects about to be covered with flaps.

to return to normal activities rather than spend another 2 or 3 months having a further reconstruction. There are certain cases, however, where such a procedure is possible and even desirable.

In conclusion, we would stress that the successful results achieved by these procedures depend, above all, on the sensibility which is preserved on the prehensile surfaces of the reconstructed digits. It is this which assures them of automatic actions and control of grip without which all efforts at reconstruction would be no better than the function provided by a prosthesis.

BIBLIOGRAPHY

ISELIN, M. (1961). Considérations sur l'amputation métacarpienne. *Mémoires de l'Académie de chirurgie*, **87,** 534–537.
ISELIN, M. & ISELIN, F. (1967). Traité de Chirurgie de la Main. *Flammarion.*
TUBIANA, R. (1958). Phalangisation du cinquième métacarpien. *Acta ortho. Belgica,* suppl, **3,** 120.

12. DIGITAL TRANSFERS AFTER AMPUTATION OF FINGERS

J-P. Razemon

Amputation of a central finger, middle or ring, results in certain inconveniences:

1. A gap is left between the remaining fingers allowing small objects to slip out even after closing the hand.
2. The stump of these amputated digits may be painful for various reasons, e.g. neuroma, vasomotor disturbances and sometimes a breakdown of the scar if this is of poor quality.
3. Lastly, there is a deviation of the main finger, index or little, the tip of which tends to incline towards the tip of the neighbouring finger. From a cosmetic point of view this is unsightly enough but this inclination also reduces the prehensile power because the tendons are deviated from their normal line of pull.

When one shakes the hand of a patient who has lost the middle or ring finger, one experiences the unpleasant sensation of a hand which becomes thin at its extremity and which tends to slip out of one's own hand.

In an attempt to overcome these inconveniences we have performed in 30 cases, a 'digital centralisation', i.e. a transfer of the main finger, index or little, on to the metacarpal of the amputated finger, middle or ring.

This results in a hand with three fingers which is narrower but has a very satisfactory appearance from the cosmetic point of view (Fig. 12.1B).

OPERATIVE TECHNIQUE

The aim is to transfer an entire finger complete with its tendons, blood supply and sensory innervation. As the amount of shift required is only of limited degree, none of these components has far to go and since most of them lie close to the palmar aspect the operation is readily carried out from the dorsum where access to bone is easy.

A racket-type incision is made around the scar of the amputated finger and extended on the dorsal aspect of the hand as far as the bases of the metacarpals to a point situated midway between the metacarpal base of the amputated finger (middle or ring) and the metacarpal base of the finger to be transferred (index or little). This approach will provide easy access to both bones which is the aim of the skeletal phase of the operation.

The operation does not present any particular difficulty but there are certain problems concerning both muscles and bones.

PROBLEMS CONCERNING THE MUSCLES

Certain of the muscles are rendered useless by the ablation of the finger to which they are attached. In amputations of the middle finger these are the 2nd and 3rd dorsal interossei and in amputations of the ring finger, the palmar interosseous of the 3rd space and the dorsal interosseous of the 4th space.

The sacrifice of these muscles is essential since transfer of the finger to its new site would otherwise involve too much useless muscle bulk and produce an unsightly prominence on the back of the hand.

The structure of these muscles is not very complicated and careful dissection going from the periphery towards their metacarpal attachments enables one to separate the palmar and dorsal interossei of the same space without difficulty. This is a simple procedure in middle finger amputations because the two dorsal interossei are readily accessible. It is slightly more difficult in ring finger amputations because in sacrificing the palmar interosseous of the 3rd space great care must be taken of the dorsal interosseous. The artery is ligated and the nerve divided at the same time as the interossei are removed.

When transferring the index finger the management of the insertion of adductor pollicis must be considered. In order to conserve the main portion of this muscle we initially divided the 3rd metacarpal at its narrowest part but this was not satisfactory for some interossei as their direction was no longer straight. Apart from this there was also some trouble with union. We now divide the metacarpal at its base. The adductor pollicis is stripped off preserving as much aponeurotic tissue as possible and in this way, we believe, the adductor of the thumb retains its normal power.

THE QUESTION OF BONY UNION

Consideration must be given to the level at which the bone is divided and the means for its fixation.

Transverse section through the middle would appear to be the simplest procedure, being relatively easy to fix at this level. Nevertheless, the entire area of bony contact is limited to the diaphyseal region and consolidation is sometimes difficult to obtain. Mortising the two bone ends together is generally very difficult to undertake and always easier to describe than to achieve. We have, therefore, abandoned attempts to obtain bony fusion in the diaphyseal region.

Transfer at the level of the distal metacarpal, as we have already seen, interferes with the action of the interosseous muscles by altering their line of pull.

We now make the transfer to the base of the metacarpal.

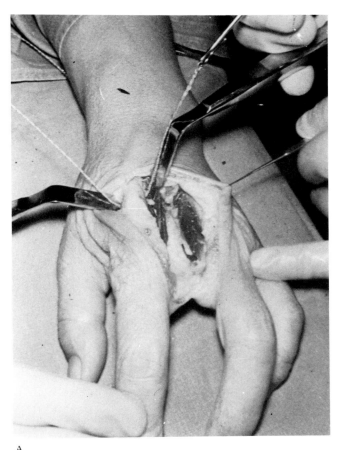

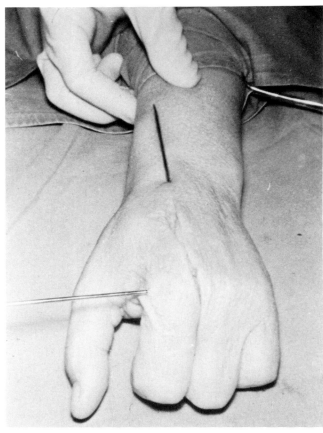

A   B

Figure 12.1

A, After removal of the middle finger stump, detachment of the interossei and section of the 3rd metacarpal at its base, the 2nd metacarpal is divided at the same level with a Gigli saw. The fibres of the 2nd and 3rd interossei, which are preserved, are seen at the site of the resected 3rd metacarpal.

B, After transposition of the index finger, fixation is secured by two Kirschner wires, a longitudinal one introduced in retrograde fashion through the transposed metacarpal and then driven into the base of the 3rd metacarpal, and a transverse one at the level of the metacarpal heads to prevent rotation. The wires are cut and buried beneath the skin.

The two metacarpals, that of the amputated finger and that of the finger to be transferred, are divided at the same level, so that the degree of tone in the tendons is not altered. The bone is divided preferably using a Gigli saw (Fig. 12.1A).

The distal part of the metacarpal of the amputated finger is removed and the detached interosseous muscles, the flexor and extensor tendons and the excess of skin are transferred. Painful neuromata are cut back as far as possible, those which are not suitable for treatment being left alone.

The transfer is easy since the space has already been prepared to receive the main finger (Fig. 12.2).

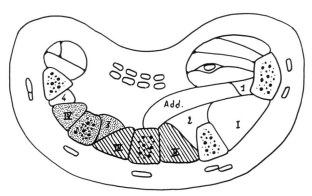

Figure 12.2

Cross section of the hand at metacarpal level. *Key:* cross hatching indicates parts resected when the index finger is transferred to the 3rd metacarpal base following amputation of the middle finger, viz., 3rd metacarpal and dorsal interossei of 2nd and 3rd spaces which are inserted into the extensor of the middle finger and are now useless; dotted areas indicate parts resected when the little finger is transferred to the 4th metacarpal base following amputation of the ring finger, viz. 4th metacarpal, the 3rd palmar and 4th dorsal interossei which are inserted into the extensor of the ring finger.

Secure skeletal fixation is achieved by two Kirschner wires. A longitudinal one is passed distally through the metacarpal of the transposed digit and out through the skin. It is then driven back into the metacarpal of the amputated digit and withdrawn proximally so that the metacarpophalangeal joint is left free. Its length is carefully calculated so that it lies as distally as possible in the metacarpal. It is cut off and buried beneath the skin at its proximal end.

For perfect fixation and, in particular, to prevent rotation, a transverse Kirschner wire is passed through the metacarpal necks which stabilises the transposed bone against its neighbour. It is introduced with the fingers in a flexed position in order to check the correct degree of rotation (Fig. 12.1B).

Fixation may also be achieved by use of a plate. This extra security enables one to dispense with plaster of Paris but it is essential to make the section through the metacarpal shaft with the disadvantages previously mentioned.

The operation is concluded by suturing the skin.

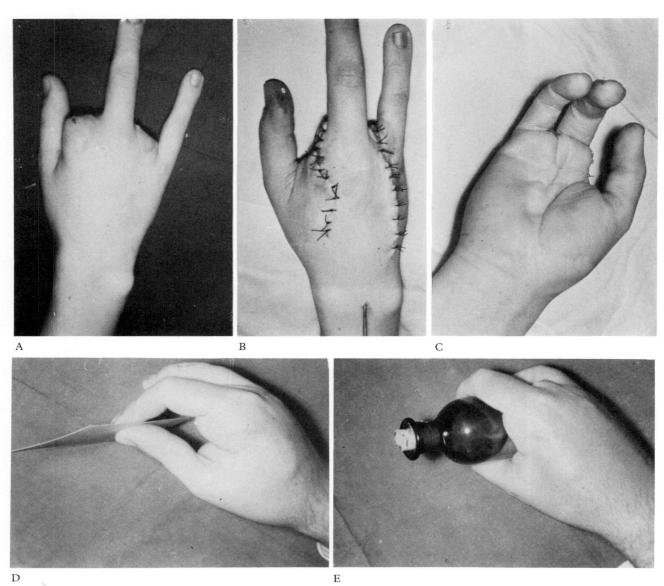

Figure 12.3
Amputations of index and ring fingers.
A, The index stump is prominent and ulcerated, the gap left after amputation of the ring finger is ugly and small objects slip out through the gap when the hand is used.
B and C, Following surgery which involved removal of the distal two-thirds of the 2nd metacarpal with transfer of the 1st dorsal interosseous on to the insertion of the 2nd and transposition of little finger to the 4th metacarpal.
D and E, Result of operation demonstrating fine and strong grip. Excellent result from both cosmetic and functional points of view.

INDICATIONS FOR DIGITAL TRANSFER

This operation is certainly not indicated in all cases of amputation of the middle or ring finger. Many patients following such injuries are quite satisfied, being able to return to normal working and have no complaints. There is no reason to intervene and necessitate their absence from work for several months by performing this reconstructive procedure.

We have been led to practise this operation in certain circumstances.

We have undertaken it on 13 occasions following amputation of the middle finger because the gain from both the cosmetic and functional points of view is assured.

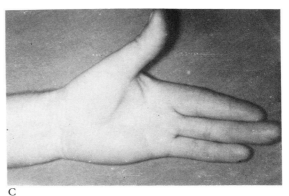

C

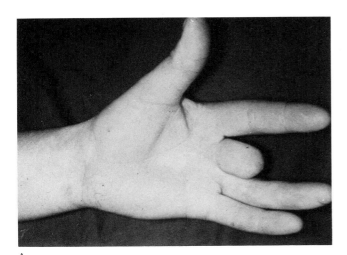

A

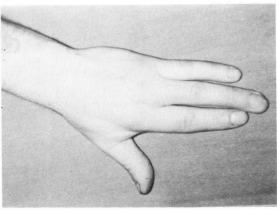

D

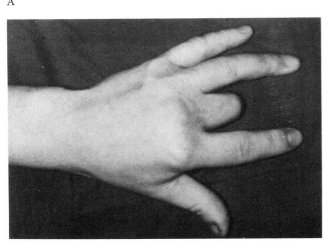

B

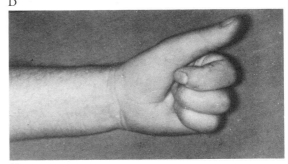

E

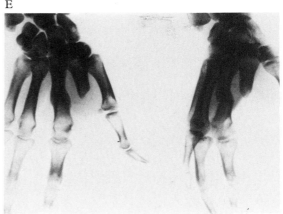

F

Figure 12.4
A and B, Painful stump of middle finger. It remains permanently flexed and being very painful to touch, makes the hand useless.
C, D, E and F, Excellent result after transfer of the middle finger to the 3rd metacarpal. The hand is no longer awkward. Function is perfect. Vasomotor disturbance and pain have disappeared. Two and a half year follow-up.

After amputation of the ring finger, however, transfer of the little finger is not nearly so easy and we have only performed it three times.

1. COSMETIC INDICATIONS

This procedure has been carried out nine times. To date we have only operated on men but it is possible that for women indications of this kind may occur more frequently. There is no doubt that transfer of the main finger to the site of an amputated middle finger gives a satisfactory cosmetic appearance to the hand. This method is, in our opinion, vastly superior to a prosthesis which cannot be functional and which is purely for show. The indications for one or other method vary and are dependent essentially on the choice of the patient. After discussing the possibilities with him one must know exactly what he himself requires before deciding whether to fit him with a prosthesis which will give a perfect cosmetic appearance but which might have to be removed for certain

jobs, or to suggest the finger transfer operation. It must be explained that this may reduce the grip but will certainly give the hand a satisfactory cosmetic appearance.

In a man who presented with amputations of index and ring fingers and in whom the stump of the index was prominent, ulcerated and painful, we carried out in a single operative procedure:

Oblique removal of the distal two-thirds of the 2nd metacarpal with re-attachment of the 1st dorsal interosseous to the tendon of the 2nd
Transfer of the little finger to the 4th metacarpal (Fig. 12.3)

2. MORE COMPLEX MUTILATIONS OF THE HAND

Digital transfer for amputation of the middle finger may, on occasion, be combined with other surgical procedures.

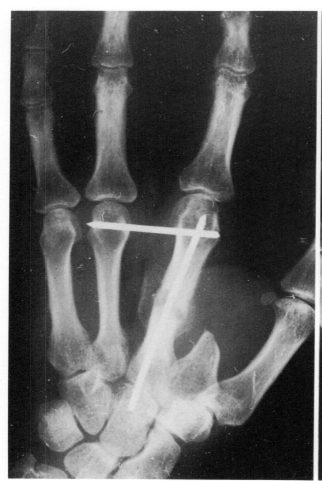 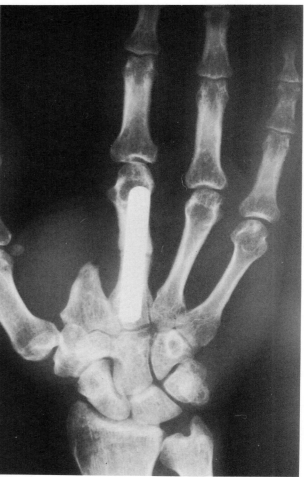

A   B

Figure 12.5
X-rays showing bone fixation.
A, With Kirschner wires.
B, With plate.

INDICATIONS FOR DIGITAL TRANSFER

This operation is certainly not indicated in all cases of amputation of the middle or ring finger. Many patients following such injuries are quite satisfied, being able to return to normal working and have no complaints. There is no reason to intervene and necessitate their absence from work for several months by performing this reconstructive procedure.

We have been led to practise this operation in certain circumstances.

We have undertaken it on 13 occasions following amputation of the middle finger because the gain from both the cosmetic and functional points of view is assured.

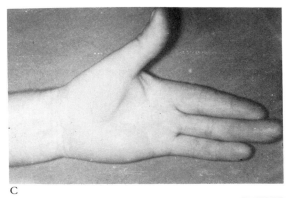
C

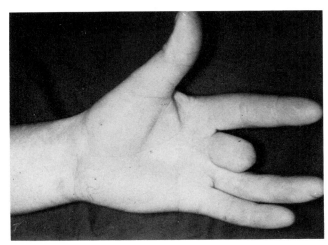
A

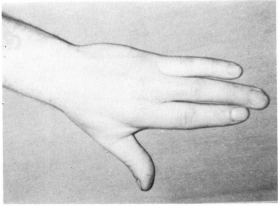
D

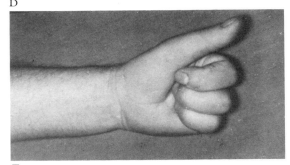
E

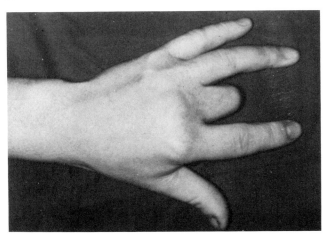
B

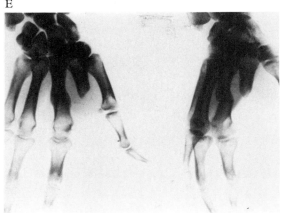
F

Figure 12.4
A and B, Painful stump of middle finger. It remains permanently flexed and being very painful to touch, makes the hand useless.
C, D, E and F, Excellent result after transfer of the middle finger to the 3rd metacarpal. The hand is no longer awkward. Function is perfect. Vasomotor disturbance and pain have disappeared. Two and a half year follow-up.

After amputation of the ring finger, however, transfer of the little finger is not nearly so easy and we have only performed it three times.

1. COSMETIC INDICATIONS

This procedure has been carried out nine times. To date we have only operated on men but it is possible that for women indications of this kind may occur more frequently. There is no doubt that transfer of the main finger to the site of an amputated middle finger gives a satisfactory cosmetic appearance. This method is, in our opinion, vastly superior to a prosthesis which cannot be functional and which is purely for show. The indications for one or other method vary and are dependent essentially on the choice of the patient. After discussing the possibilities with him one must know exactly what he himself requires before deciding whether to fit him with a prosthesis which will give a perfect cosmetic appearance but which might have to be removed for certain jobs, or to suggest the finger transfer operation. It must be explained that this may reduce the grip but will certainly give the hand a satisfactory cosmetic appearance.

In a man who presented with amputations of index and ring fingers and in whom the stump of the index was prominent, ulcerated and painful, we carried out in a single operative procedure:

Oblique removal of the distal two-thirds of the 2nd metacarpal with re-attachment of the 1st dorsal interosseous to the tendon of the 2nd
Transfer of the little finger to the 4th metacarpal (Fig. 12.3)

2. MORE COMPLEX MUTILATIONS OF THE HAND

Digital transfer for amputation of the middle finger may, on occasion, be combined with other surgical procedures.

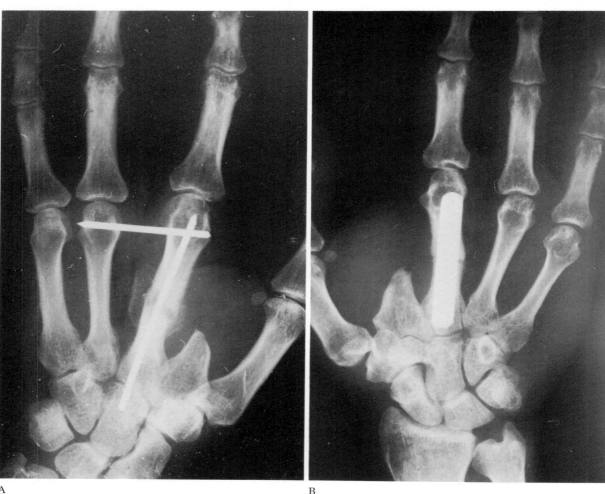

A   B

Figure 12.5
X-rays showing bone fixation.
A, With Kirschner wires.
B, With plate.

This was the case in one patient who presented with an amputation of the middle finger, malunion of the proximal phalanx of the index finger with considerable angulation and a fixed adduction deformity of the thumb in addition to complications following fractures of both its phalanges. In one operative procedure we corrected the adduction deformity of the thumb by a Z-plasty and removal of the fibrous tissue from the first web, adjusted the angulation deformity of the index finger by osteotomy and pin fixation and transferred the index finger to the 3rd metacarpal.

3. A COMPLEMENTARY PROCEDURE TO POLLICISATION

The gap left after utilisation of a finger to replace an absent thumb may be closed by transferring an adjacent finger to the remaining metacarpal and this improves the cosmetic appearance of the hand.

4. VASOMOTOR PROBLEMS AND PAINFUL FINGER STUMPS

The final indication has produced results of particular interest. Painful amputation stumps and vasomotor disturbances are not infrequent particularly when there is a poor scar and an unsightly gap. It occurred to us that, rather than tackling the neuroma in the stump or more proximally, it would be of interest to remove this abnormal stump which, by its very presence, certainly causes functional and psychological disturbances seen in such patients.

Transfer of the index finger removes the abnormal space resulting from amputation of the middle finger. The patient is no longer able to see the offending stump and this is a most important factor in his cure. We have carried out this procedure on five painful stumps, all middle finger ones. Four of these were available for assessment. The results have been particularly impressive because the patients have been literally cured of their painful stumps. This suggests that a physiopathological study might be made into the origin of these complications following amputation, with advantage. Whilst not claiming to have given the patient back a normal hand, there is no doubt that the cosmetic appearance is satisfactory and the patient is no longer squeamish about it (Fig. 12.4). He does not now consider himself mutilated and this contributes much to his rehabilitation.

CONCLUSION

Transfer of the index finger to the metacarpal of an amputated middle finger is a reconstructive procedure which has undoubted cosmetic value, but the most interesting aspect has emerged in the way that painful middle finger stumps have been cured by this transfer.

Removal of the abnormal stump corrects both the psychological disturbances and the loss of functioning ability resulting from amputation.

13. RECONSTRUCTION OF THE AMPUTATED THUMB

J. Gosset

We are not concerned here with problems presented by congenital malformation of the hand, where the thumb may be absent or represented only by a vestigial element lacking function or having the characteristics of a finger (the triphalangeal thumb) which has no opposition function. The latter is the so-called five-fingered hand.

These congenital malformations only have a relative reduction of functional capacity. The affected children learn from an early age to use these abnormal hands. Their appearance differs from that of the normal hand but they use them with facility. Indications for surgical correction stem less from functional considerations than from social, cosmetic and psychological considerations raised by the parents. The child himself only becomes aware of his deformity at school age but it is advisable to operate before this, at an age before mechanisms of prehension have become firmly established.

In the adult, we are only concerned with traumatic amputations. Indications for reconstruction of the thumb must be carefully weighed. The question whether to operate and the choice of operation will be discussed more than the actual techniques of surgical reconstruction which are today generally well established. Only certain details of technique merit further research and slight improvement.

In our opinion, one should accept for operation only those patients who ask for reconstruction or freely accept advice to have an operation. The successes of organ transplantation have been extolled so freely in the press that many patients imagine that one can graft on a cadaver thumb. They are disillusioned when informed of the actual situation. It is easy to convince a patient of the value of a Gillies' lengthening operation or phalangisation, in limited distal amputations. They will usually accept (and, in our opinion, quite wrongly) the Nicoladoni tubed flap reconstruction. On the other hand, in many instances, they do not readily accept the principle of a digital transfer. This is the case with the skilled worker who accepts a hand deprived of thumb/finger opposition, i.e. a hand which can only be used as a hook with limited grasping ability. This also applies in the adolescent when the parents refuse operation because they fail to understand the advantages or to appreciate the results which may be achieved. The long-standing amputee is less likely to agree to reconstruction. We do not attempt to persuade patients to undergo reconstructive procedures. The psychological attitude of the patient is, in our view, of prime importance in his rehabilitation and training to use the new thumb. The patient's will for recovery is so important that reconstruction is not attempted in those who have too readily accepted their disability. Lethargic, frightened or passive individuals prefer to accept their disability than to make the effort that rehabilitation requires. Moreover, they fear (wrongly) that a thumb reconstruction will reduce their disability allowance which they would prefer to be increased.

In some cases, our confidence in being able to help these amputees has led us to try to influence them by showing them other cases where reconstruction has been undertaken. Our reticence in this respect has perhaps been excessive as demonstrated by the following two cases. A 40-year old man, having lost the right thumb at 18, approached us with a request to be fitted with a plastic prosthesis for cosmetic reasons. We agreed to this whilst, at the same time, pointing out that we should only have considered suggesting digital transfer had the thumb loss been a more recent occurrence. He demanded operation, which we undertook, and this was highly successful.

The second case concerned a North African workman. As far as we could judge the prognosis for reconstruction in his case was poor because of his psychological state. We were mistaken because he proved to be one of the few patients who has shown both a desire to recover and exceptional skill with his new thumb.

This preoperative psychological assessment seems to us to be indispensable. It is often worthwhile to have the expert advice of a specialist in psychological medicine.

We have never used a digital transfer for phalangeal losses. In these cases, the Gillies' lengthening operation, with or without deepening of the web, is generally adequate both from functional and cosmetic points of view.

In our opinion, reconstruction of the thumb amputated through the first metacarpal is only justifiable if it guarantees an excellent functional and cosmetic result. The new thumb must have a more or less normal appearance with restoration of the lateral pinch, pulp to pulp pinch and a powerful grasp. This is why, as a means of thumb reconstruction, we are against the Nicoladoni-type operation. Reconstituting the thumb by means of a skin tube creates at best an insensitive cylindrical buffer which is unsightly and easily traumatised. Moreover, this sort of result is achieved only by multiple operations. Complications are more frequent than is generally acknowledged.

Multiple operative procedures, in addition to involving prolonged incapacity, may sometimes cause serious psychological disturbances. We recall a young woman who, having undergone eight operations by an experienced surgeon, came and begged us to remove a painful, useless stump the appearance of which was abhorrent to her. How many long and ambitious tubes have been shortened following terminal necrosis? How many bone grafts have been absorbed, fractured or disintegrated by osteitis following minimal infection of the extremity of the tube? We have had occasion to examine a number of thumbs reconstructed elsewhere by such a procedure. The new thumb appeared short, swollen and sausage-like. If the bone graft was long, it undermined the viability of the skin. If there was surplus skin, the end of the stump was flabby, mobile and failed to provide adequate pinch or power grip. A cyanotic tinge to the end of the tube indicated its precarious circulation and thus the vulnerability of the new thumb. From neither the cosmetic nor the functional point of view could these thumbs be compared with the results of digital transfers. Lack of sensation in the reconstructed thumb by the Nicoladoni procedure has appeared to justify a complementary operation, i.e. transfer of a neurovascular island flap. This operation is almost as complicated as a total digital transfer.

Whilst we are able to quote important statistics concerning digital transfers (Littler, Buck-Gramcko, Harrison, etc.) we have not found any concerning the Nicoladoni operation.

Being aware of the fact that certain advocates of the use of the tubed flap, bone graft procedure are resolutely opposed to pollicisation by the transfer of an intact finger, we feel this to be the only defensible technique.

The pros and cons must be discussed. They concern two different kinds of case: where there is an isolated amputation of the thumb and where several remaining fingers have been mutilated.

In the first group (four intact fingers) those who oppose pollicisation argue that it is not justifiable to 'sacrifice' a normal finger to remake a thumb. Everything turns on the significance of the term 'sacrifice'. If pollicisation presented real risks, e.g. necrosis and loss of the new thumb, the argument against it would be admissible. This is not so, however, since we have never observed loss, even partial, following transfer of a healthy finger. The blood supply of the finger is remarkable as we demonstrated in a single case where a surgical error was committed. We made a careless blunder whilst cutting through the base of the proximal phalanx dividing the neurovascular bundle which had been inadequately protected. The nerve was repaired and the artery tied. There was no further difficulty and the functional result was excellent. We do not claim that a single vascular pedicle should always be sufficient. In this instance there was almost certainly a deep palmar branch which enhanced the blood supply.

A pollicised finger is never just a sacrificed one. The patient only ever has just the four fingers but the value of one of these has been increased. In the words of Littler the operation increases the strategic value of the transferred finger. One can produce numerical proof of this. According to Swanson, if one gives the five digits an overall value of one hundred, the thumb counts as 40 per cent, the index and middle fingers as 20 per cent each and the ring and little fingers as 10 per cent each. Personally, we feel that the little finger is of greater value than the ring finger for a strong grasp. We are therefore, inclined to rate the ring finger as 7 per cent and the little finger as 13 per cent.

Adhering to Swanson's evaluation, a thumbless hand with four intact fingers is worth 60. After pollicisation of the ring finger it is worth 90, i.e. a 30 per cent gain on the original state.

There is another argument presented by the opponents of pollicisation namely that the subject will not use his new thumb. They believe the latter will be purely cosmetic and the hand will possess only three useful fingers. This opinion is quite contrary to the results we have observed in our patients, whether it be in a professional person or a workman. They use their new thumb well for opposition in fine manipulations or power grip at work as well as for everyday use.

The other group is where the thumb has been amputated and one or more fingers have been mutilated. If the mutilations affect two or three of the remaining fingers and are severe with, for example, partial amputations, joint injuries, tendon lesions and divisions of nerves, one enters the field of an atypical reconstruction where there can be no fixed rule or guiding principle. One looks for the most suitable stump to make an opposable thumb and, not unnaturally, one leaves the first or the sound fingers in place. Each case thus poses a particular problem. One does not consider the cosmetic aspect. We are only concerned with function. This varies from case to case depending on the individual's work and the functional potential remaining. If he has an adequate grasp more is gained by fitting a prosthesis rather than attempting surgical reconstruction. If grasp is lacking one can often recreate a pinch by metacarpal phalangisation with or without transfer of a metacarpal base. The description of these atypical procedures which we have carried out on a few occasions should emerge from the substance of this account although they cannot be classified.

We must now discuss mutilation of a single finger and it is frequently the index. Again using the term 'sacrifice', certain authorities feel that it is better to sacrifice an already mutilated finger. We do not agree with this. It is our opinion, that to re-make a cosmetic and functional thumb it is preferable and more certain to use the best available material, i.e. a sound finger. Much depends on the degree of mutilation. The work of Roullet seems to us very significant in this respect. The latter has considered particularly the case of a neurovascular injury to the index finger associated with loss of the thumb. Using an original technique to transfer the entire index finger with its interossei, Roullet preserves the important blood supply in the index which stems from the anastomosis between the interosseal artery and the digital artery. The procedure is claimed to be a satisfactory one. We, however, are not convinced that transfer of the ring finger followed by suture of the digital nerves of the index would not be equivalent. Removal of the index finger, on the other hand, reduces the breadth of the palm much more than is the case with either middle or ring fingers. Lastly, opposition of the new thumb to the middle finger provides a greater range of movement than opposition achieved by a pollicised index finger.

Based on our experience of 27 pollicisations using the Hilgenfeldt technique which presented no problems, we shall now describe our own method. It differs from Hilgenfeldt's

F

only in that we prefer to use the ring finger rather than the middle.

Transfer of the middle finger leaves an unsightly gap between the index and ring fingers if one conserves the head of the 3rd metacarpal. If one sacrifices it, one removes the central pillar of the hand and there is a risk of the ring finger rotating. From the anatomical point of view, transfer of the middle finger slackens the flexor tendons. Hilgenfeldt has noticed this since he advocates a tendon shortening procedure in the forearm which we have also had to do in our only middle finger transfer. The ring finger, however, is far enough away from the thumb for its transfer not to interfere with normal tension in the flexor tendons.

The age of the patient is not of any great significance. Our patients ranged in age from 17 to 52 years. However, we should not envisage such a procedure in patients over 60 or under 12 years of age. Within these limits, the young will recover more quickly than the old and our best result was in a 17-year old boy. Naturally, this reconstruction would be contra-indicated in severe arthritis or in patients with vascular disturbances: Raynaud's disease, acrocyanosis, Buerger's disease, localised arteritis following frostbite.

It remains to discuss the timing of operation. We feel it is best done shortly after amputation. On one occasion, we undertook it before the amputation site had healed.

Pollicisation must be delayed, however, if skin loss or scarring of the thenar region requires some form of skin replacement preferably with a pedicle flap.

All our cases except four had sustained traumatic amputation of the thumb. In these four cases, where we had to amputate the thumb for some other reason we did a pollicisation at the same time by transferring the ring finger.

The first of these cases was a garage mechanic who sustained an oil injection injury when a jet of oil under high pressure accidentally entered his thumb. Attempts to cure the resulting oleoma by repeated operations failed. The thumb was red, had multiple sinuses and was stiff. Amputation was the only effective treatment available. The sinuses were found to extend as far as the flexor tendon sheath. The result following pollicisation of the ring finger was so perfect that the patient was able to carry out without difficulty all his work as a mechanic from the most delicate manipulations to the heaviest tasks. The other three cases were patients with malignant melanomata of the thumb. The functional results were excellent. One of them has been lost to follow-up. Another is well after 16 years. The remaining one was treated only two years ago. In two out of the three cases pollicisation was combined by a block dissection of the axilla.

TECHNIQUE

The operation is carried out under general anaesthesia and in a bloodless field. Its duration scarcely exceeds, in general, the time for which the pneumatic tourniquet is kept in place. After an hour and a quarter all the delicate steps of the operation have been completed. Removal of the tourniquet at this stage is not accompanied by any appreciable bleeding nor does it interfere with completion of the operation.

EXCISION OF THE AMPUTATION SCAR

This excision removes all the scar tissue but conserves the maximum of healthy tissue. It removes a circular area from the end of the stump. This is extended by a vertical dorsal dissection of 3 to 4 centimetres in the line of the metacarpal. This dissection is to expose the extensor tendons. Into this space will be placed the small triangular dorsal flap cut from the ring finger distal to the metacarpophalangeal joint.

THE PALMAR INCISIONS

There are three palmar incisions which are made at once, incising skin only. Two of these incisions form a V at an angle of about 90°. One of the branches of this follows the longitudinal line of the 3rd intermetacarpal space between the middle and ring fingers to a point situated in the middle of the palm at the distal border of the flexor retinaculum. It must be remembered that this edge of the flexor retinaculum lies about 5 cm beyond the distal flexion crease of the wrist. This lower edge is in line with the ulnar border of the proximal phalanx of the normal thumb when it is held in full abduction. There is reason for this incision to be very slightly inclined and within the axis of the intermetacarpal space, a little nearer the ring finger than the middle. This is to facilitate the skin suture at the end of operation. The other branch of the V is dissected from the proximal end of the intermetacarpal incision towards a point which would correspond with the interval between the sesamoid bones of the thumb. It then follows the line of the flexor tendon of the thumb. The two branches are an average of 6 cm in length and, above all, are of equal length, these distances being measured from the apex of the V to the middle/ring web on one side and to the metacarpophalangeal palmar skinfold of the thumb on the other (or at least to the site where this crease would have been if the thumb had not been amputated).

The other palmar incision starts at the web between the ring and little fingers, extends the length of the 4th intermetacarpal space inclining very slightly radially towards the ring finger. In the proximal palm, it ends at a level slightly distal to the apex of the V previously described (5 mm more distally).

The two parallel intermetacarpal incisions are separated by about 10 to 11 mm.

We wish to stress the importance initially of making nothing but superficial incisions, incising only the skin and never involving the palmar aponeurosis at this stage.

EXPOSURE OF THE THENAR EMINENCE

The thenar eminence is approached through the radial limb of the V previously described. Sharp scalpel dissection is used initially but then short curved scissors are more useful for deepening the incision. The thenar muscles are left intact and one seeks to isolate the distal end of the 1st metacarpal. Sometimes amputation occurs at the metacarpophalangeal joint. The head of the metacarpal remains and even the sesamoids, which are removed. In other cases amputation is more proximal through the neck, the shaft or even the base of the 1st metacarpal. One again looks for the end of the bone.

It is cleared by scalpel dissection or stripped with a periosteal elevator for a distance of 2 cm.

Before making what we shall call 'the preparation of the 1st metacarpal' one looks for neuromata of the digital nerves. These two nerves are isolated by dissection. The neuromata are resected and the nerve trunks are then diathermised using the technique advocated by us to avoid recurrence of neuromata. None of our patients has complained of thenar pain due to neuroma formation after thumb reconstruction.

One now looks for flexor pollicis longus which lies more deeply and in the median axis of the thenar eminence. Its stump is freed and the tendon cut right back. Rightly or wrongly, we have never considered using the flexor tendon of the thumb in the course of a pollicisation. Re-attachment to one of the flexors of the transferred digit in the depths of the thumb region could lead to adhesion formation. This re-attachment should only be made if the need arises as a secondary procedure and then the suture should be made at wrist level.

One then turns to the back of the thumb to find the divided ends of the two extensor tendons. One may extend the incision proximally from the point of the dorsal V, outlined at the time when the amputation scar was excised, should the extensor tendon have retracted. To date, we have always found these tendons without difficulty.

In those rare cases of thumb avulsion (and not section) the tendons will have been torn off at their junction with muscle bellies. The extensor indicis proprius could then be used to replace them.

PREPARATION OF THE 1st METACARPAL

The 1st metacarpal must now be prepared to receive the proximal phalanx of the transposed ring finger. This latter will be bevelled at the end. It is necessary to fashion a mortise in the 1st metacarpal. The most useful instrument for this purpose is the circular saw driven by a dental engine. One begins by sectioning the 1st metacarpal strictly at right angles to its axis. One must decide where to make this cut. The ideal place is at the junction of its proximal two-thirds with its distal third, i.e. about 3 cm beyond the carpo-metacarpal joint. If the thumb has been amputated through the midshaft of the 1st metacarpal, all one can do is carefully to fashion the end of the bone. Still greater care must be taken should the amputation site be proximal to this or even at the metacarpal base. In this event, it is prepared with bone nibblers to freshen its end so that the short metacarpal stump will have a satisfactory surface. Later, we shall discuss management of total loss of the 1st metacarpal at its articulation with the trapezium.

In most cases, thumb loss has occurred at a distal level, sometimes even through the metacarpophalangeal joint. In these cases there is a strong tendency to leave too great a metacarpal length. Three centimetres of metacarpal beyond the carpometacarpal joint are quite sufficient. The two sides of the slot forming the mortise are always fashioned with the saw. One must remember that the 1st metacarpal is flattened with a convex dorsal surface and a flat or even slightly concave

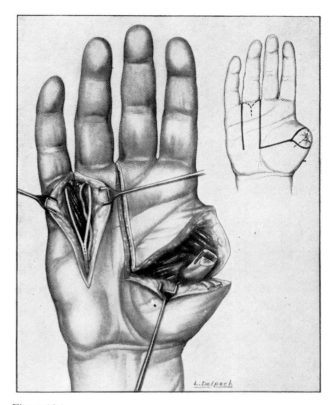

Figure 13.1
Incisions outlined. Neurovascular bundles displayed. Preparation of 1st metacarpal.

palmar aspect with two borders one on the ulnar edge, the other on the radial. The level of section must be equidistant from the metacarpal axis and, as a general principle, strictly at right angles to the surface joining the two edges of the metacarpal. The slot made by the saw must be 12 to 13 mm deep. The two edges are separated by about 5 mm. With a fine gouge the bony fragments are removed from the slot created by the saw cuts. By this means a sagittal defect is made at the metacarpal end with bony prolongations on either side about 4 mm thick since they include the cortical bone.

When the bevelled end of the proximal phalanx of the ring finger is introduced into the mortise, provided that the dorsal aspects of both the 1st metacarpal and the proximal phalanx of the pollicised finger are in the same plane, the transferred finger will be in the exact position necessary for normal opposition.

This ideal state of affairs is not always realised. It may happen following amputation of the thumb, with a prolonged period of immobilisation in a bad position, that fibrosis of the muscles of the first web space together with some stiffening of the metacarpophalangeal joint will have reduced the opposition range of the 1st metacarpal. When this is the case, the palmar aspect of the 1st metacarpal faces forward too much in maximal opposition. If one strictly adhered to the rule which we are about to formulate, the new thumb should provide a pinch with the index and middle fingers using only the ulnar aspect of its distal phalanx instead of the whole pulp. In these cases, which form a minority, the slot must be cut obliquely in relationship to the axis of the first metacarpal. On the dorsum the radial boundary becomes larger than the ulnar. Inversely, on the palmar aspect, the ulnar boundary is larger than the radial.

ISOLATION OF THE NEUROVASCULAR BUNDLES OF THE 3rd AND 4th INTERMETACARPAL SPACES

The aim of this dissection is to preserve the blood supply and the innervation of the finger to be pollicised. The innervation includes the digital nerve to the ulnar side of the 3rd space and the digital nerve to the radial side of the 4th space. From the vascular point of view, these are all the digital arteries which must be taken with the finger to be transferred. This means that the collateral branches to the ulnar side of the middle finger and the radial side of the little finger, must be ligated and divided. In each of the metacarpal incisions the surgical procedures are as follows: one carefully incises the palmar aponeurosis which in a normal hand is very thin being rather like trellis work. It may even be absent in the distal part of the space. This exposes the neurovascular bundles which must be dissected from the proximal part of the incision in a distal direction taking care not to injure the vessels, particularly the veins. The nerves should be dissected first.

The division of the common volar digital nerve into its two collateral branches occurs at a variable level. It is of little consequence. The two branches must be dissected from a distal level in a proximal direction so that they are completely separated one from the other to the level of the proximal extremity of the palmar incision. There is no difficulty about this. With a scalpel one frees the perineurium and the nerves are readily separated to the proximal part of the incision. In rare instances the nerve forms a loop around the artery. This would not prove troublesome if the loop, located in the 3rd space, involves the fibres supplying the middle finger, or in the 4th space, the nerve fibres going to the little finger. This would simply require further separation of the nerve to a more proximal level. Then, only the arteriovenous bundle has to be dealt with. The artery is divided in Y widely open, very distally just at the level of the web. The disssection of this bifurcation must be done very gently because tearing would be disastrous. In the 3rd space, one dissects a good centimetre from the digital vessel to the ulnar side of the middle finger. It is divided between two ligatures taking great care that the proximal ligature is not placed too near the bifurcation. This precaution is essential to avoid any interference with the blood supply of the finger to be transferred. In the 4th space it is the digital vessel to the radial side of the little finger which has to be ligated in the same way. After this, constant care has to be taken to visualise the neurovascular bundles which have been dissected. They must be gently retracted with a blunt hook so they are not at risk in the course of subsequent procedures.

Before turning to the dorsal procedure, all that remains is to divide the vertical extensions of the palmar aponeurosis in front of the interosseous muscles and also to divide the latter slightly.

We have twice met with a tiresome arterial anomaly. The digital artery in the 4th space was too short. It arose from the deep palmar arch and emerged vertically across the interosseous muscles. We feared then that transfer of the finger would stretch it dangerously. By basing it far towards the distal end of the intermetacarpal space we were able to free it sufficiently to prevent any untoward incident.

DORSAL PROCEDURE

The two palmar skin incisions are extended around the base of the finger on to the dorsal aspect where they join in a racket fashion forming a short V. The point of the V is situated just proximal to the level of the joint. The dorsal vessels on either side are ligated and divided. The extensor tendon is cut at a more proximal level. It is then dissected, working from above downwards, from the head of the metacarpal and the base of the proximal phalanx.

The lateral extensions of the interossei are carefully dissected free, isolated and divided leaving as much length as possible from their attachments to the distal end of the extensor tendon. One then proceeds to disarticulate the metacarpophalangeal joint. The dorsal capsule, both collateral ligaments and anterior capsule are divided in turn. This procedure must be undertaken with care, the assistant visualising and protecting with retractors throughout the neurovascular bundles already dissected in the palmar procedure.

The disarticulated ring finger now remains attached to the palm by two freely mobilised neurovascular bundles, a narrow skin strip covering both flexor tendons which have not been seen until now. These tendons remain in the depths, held in close contact with the 4th metacarpal by the fibrous sheath and the vertical fibres of the palmar aponeurosis. It now remains to divide these attachments in the final mobilisation of the finger to leave a cutaneous-neurovascular-tendinous pedicle at the proximal part of the palm.

Flexing the finger towards the palm, one works from the dorsal aspect on the deep surface of flexor profundus dividing on its two edges all the tissues which keep it tethered. This freeing is essential and must be extended proximally as far as the level of the skin pedicle, i.e. to the level of the distal edge of the flexor retinaculum. There is no doubt that in our early cases we did not carry out this procedure as thoroughly as we should have done. The finger having been transferred, the flexor tendons took an angled course whilst held by the remaining fibrous elements in the line of the 4th metacarpal. This must be avoided if one wishes to maintain effective action on the pollicised finger. During this procedure, it is also necessary to detach the lumbricals whose common attachments would continue to link the flexor profundus of the ring finger to that of the adjacent flexor.

Harrison, in the meeting of the Groupe d'Etude de la Main of 21 November 1967, advised division of the flexor superficialis of the transferred finger and its re-attachment for opposition on the side of the new metacarpophalangeal joint (proximal interphalangeal joint of the transferred finger). One must then continue the incision to the wrist so that palmaris longus serves as a pulley for the flexor superficialis. Theoretically, this is a logical idea for a normal thumb has only one flexor tendon. However, following pollicisation opposition is always strong. We have been anxious to adhere to Hilgenfeldt's operation in principle. This necessitates keeping the combined skin-tendinous pedicle intact so as not to interfere with its gliding properties. For this reason therefore, we have not followed Harrison's suggestion. Moreover, Harrison recognises that his procedure could create a swan neck deformity of the new thumb.

PREPARATION OF THE PROXIMAL PHALANX OF THE RING FINGER

The base of the proximal phalanx of the ring finger is held in a small Farabeuf's forceps. Using a scalpel rather than a rugine one frees the bone for a good 2 cm. On the sides of the palmar aspect of the phalanx, one divides the phalangeal attachment of the fibrous sheath. With great care, using a very small circular saw or a dental burr, the cartilage is scraped off the phalangeal base or, preferably, using the saw 2 mm may be removed from the base cutting parallel to its surface. Two sagittal cuts accurately placed 5 mm apart are now made with the saw to correspond with the width of the mortise in the first metacarpal. The length of this peg must also be equivalent to the depth of the mortise. The lateral edges of the phalanx are trimmed off in fashioning the peg. The peg must be neither too wide nor too narrow. If it is too narrow, there will be play in the metacarpal slot. If it is too wide, the edges of the mortise may be ruptured whilst trying to force it in. It is essential that its edges are strictly parallel so that it does not slip out distally. It is better to cut it a little too broad and reduce it later with the dental burr, to the necessary fit when preparing the mortise in the 1st metacarpal.

INSERTION OF THE PHALANGEAL PEG OF THE RING FINGER INTO THE METACARPAL MORTISE

The isolated ring finger, lifted towards the palm, is rotated radially so that all the soft parts which form its pedicle are lying in the muscular furrow prepared in the line of the thenar eminence. This furrow must be sufficiently deep and wide to enable the vessels and tendons of the ring finger to lie comfortably in it. The peg is introduced into its mortise. It must fit closely but without having to force it in. A final reduction of either the peg or the mortise with the burr may be necessary at this point.

Sometimes, the mortise is not deep enough. In this case, one removes a little cortical bone from either the dorsal or palmar aspect of the mortise in the metacarpal with a narrow gouge. The proximal phalanx being thicker than the broad and flattened 1st metacarpal, the cortex of the phalanx will always overlap on the palmar aspect of the metacarpal because it must be arranged that the dorsal aspects of the two bones are in the same plane.

The position of the pollicised finger will also be checked. Provided the bones have been correctly cut, the new thumb should immediately assume the position of normal opposition. It would be unfortunate if an initial surgical error had been made because any alterations at this stage, which is always possible, would adversely affect the strength of the mortise joint.

This fixation is normally sufficiently strong not to require reinforcement by circumferential wiring or a Kirschner wire.

During suture of the soft tissues and plastering, there is virtually no risk of secondary displacement.

Should the mortise joint be too slack with risk of displacement, a Kirschner wire may be introduced in the proximal phalanx in retrograde fashion and then driven into the metacarpal and out through the skin. It is withdrawn at the end of the operation once the plaster has set.

The placing of a pin to remain in place for 20 to 25 days is justified only in cases where either little or none of the metacarpal remains.

In the first case, where a centimetre or so of the metacarpal base remains, the proximal phalanx may be driven into this spongy base which is often friable and decalcified, and fixation is maintained by a centrally placed pin entering the trapezium. The pin emerges on the back of the pollicised finger at the level of the head of the proximal phalanx. In fact, it passes through the extensor tendon without causing any trouble.

Where the whole of the 1st metacarpal is absent, the cartilage could be removed from the distal surface of the trapezium with bone nibblers. One does not aim to embed the proximal phalanx of the ring finger in the trapezium, as this would create an arthrodesis, which is to be avoided. Instead, the whole base of the proximal phalanx of the ring finger should be preserved together with a fringe of capsule. This is sutured to the ligamentous tissues around the trapezium. A Kirschner wire is driven through the phalanx into the trapezium roughly approximating the two bones. A fibrous pseudarthrosis will result similar to that which occurs after the operation of removal of the trapezium for arthritis of the carpometacarpal joint of the thumb. Two of our cases required this technique and excellent mobility resulted in the thumb. It was impossible however, to re-attach the long abductor to the base of the proximal phalanx.

There are other means available for total loss of the 1st metacarpal. These have been described by Buck-Gramcko and Harrison but only in reconstruction of congenital agenesis of the thumb in the child. Should they be applied in cases of traumatic loss? We have no experience of them. These two procedures use the metacarpophalangeal joint of the pollicised finger, preoperative X-rays having shown complete absence of the metacarpal. Instead of disarticulating the finger to be transferred, at the metacarpophalangeal joint, it is divided through the neck of the metacarpal.

Harrison bevels the metacarpal fragment and fixes it with stainless steel wire to the freshened base of the second metacarpal. Buck-Gramcko resects the metacarpal neck to the level of the cartilage and fixes the metacarpal head into the trapezometacarpal angle with two crossed metal pins. In the child, any hyperextension at this new trapezometacarpal joint would be troublesome. One way of overcoming this would be to perform an anterior capsulorrhaphy of the metacarpo-phalangeal joint of the pollicised finger by the Zancolli method.

We now feel we have available a possible and simpler technique which could be used for cases with total loss of thumb metacarpal. We suggest preparing the articular surface of the trapezium with the burr and then reaming out two tunnels, one in the canal of the proximal phalanx and the other in the trapezium and as far as the scaphoid. A Swanson silicone prosthesis could then be introduced simultaneously into the phalanx and the trapezium which should ensure a supple and stable joint. We intend to try out this method in our next suitable case.

CONTROL OF THE VIABILITY OF THE POLLICISED DIGIT

Before suturing the extensor tendons and the skin, the tourniquet is released and removed. It is essential to ensure strict haemostasis and make sure that the blood supply of the pollicised finger is good. As a rule, it is only necessary to tie two or three bleeding points in the distal part of the thenar

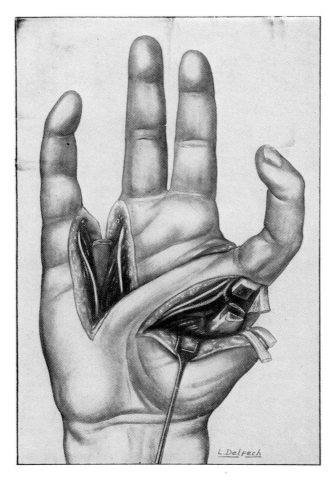

Figure 12.3
Transfer of ring finger. Note removal of head of 4th metacarpal.

eminence but very rarely a vessel arising from the deep palmar arch in the 4th space. On one occasion, suction drainage for 48 hours was used, because of persistent oozing from the thenar region.

The colour of the pollicised finger is checked. Usually, the colour returns within 2 to 3 seconds following release of the tourniquet. Sometimes it may take 30 to 60 seconds if the operation has produced vasospasm of the mobilised digital vessels. Exceptionally, the digit will remain paler than the rest of the hand until the end of operation. In this case, the first thing to do is to check that there is no kinking or abnormal tension on the vascular pedicle. Sometimes it is necessary to divide a small fibrous band or to deepen the thenar bed. In spite of this, in two of our cases, at the end of operation, the finger remained very pale and caused considerable concern. The plaster, of course, never completely covers the end of the pollicised digit so that it is possible to keep a close watch on its appearance postoperatively. In these two cases, everything had returned to normal again in less than 6 hours. Is there a case for the use of injections or a stellate ganglion block in such instances? They cause no harm and are worth trying. For our part, provided we are sure that one of the palmar digital vessels has not been damaged, such an incident does not worry us unduly since it has never led to troublesome consequences. Much more alarming, would be a purplish cyanosed appearance of the digit. This would indicate an inadequate venous return with a very grave prognosis. Necrosis, possibly of limited degree, is a potential complication. This happened in one of our cases, viz., transfer of a mutilated middle finger. Only the extremity of the finger had to be sacrificed, the remaining part surviving by the use of a pedicle flap.

RE-INSERTION OF THE EXTENSOR TENDONS AND SKIN CLOSURE

In all our cases, except two, we have been able to find both extensor tendons of the thumb. In the two exceptions only one tendon remained. We have never had to undertake a tendon transfer, which incidentally would be a simple matter, extensor indicis being readily available. The extensor tendons are re-attached in the Pulvertaft manner to the extensor of the ring finger. There is one important technical point. Should the suture be made only to the ulnar band, there would be insufficient extension of the terminal phalanx. The attachment must therefore be done simultaneously to the ulnar band and to the fibres of insertion of the interosseous on the radial side which have been dissected, and divided sufficiently proximal. There must be adequate tension in the extensor tendon but not such as to hinder the action of the flexors. This is a question of judgement which only comes with experience. We have never re-attached the thenar muscles or what remains of them and yet the movements of adduction and opposition of the new thumb have been those in which the most perfect recovery has occurred. There is no doubt that the flexors of the pollicised digit contribute to this opposition.

The skin closure presents no difficulty: the circumference of the base of the ring finger is sutured to the edges of the circular excision of the old scar. The palmar skin strip is sutured to the sides of the thenar defect. Closure of the gap left by removal of the ring finger is always easy. We use a loose suture through the nail which will bind the new thumb to the index and middle fingers. This prevents any risk of secondary displacement. Slight compression is provided with a well moulded plaster which immobilises the hand but leaves the terminal phalanx of the new thumb and the distal two phalanges of the other three fingers free. There has never been any postoperative infection. From the first week, the patient is encouraged to move the index, middle and little fingers. It may be observed that, as a rule, he is able to produce slight movements of the terminal phalanx of the thumb.

The plaster is removed on the twenty-first day when the sutures are also removed. Should a Kirschner wire have been used, it is extracted at this stage.

Active rehabilitation is started with regular daily sessions. Two hours a day are devoted to this until the patient resumes work. This varies from $2\frac{1}{2}$ to 4 months after operation. Occupational therapy is equally important. The ideal, at which we aim for each patient, is to give him an incentive to obtain promotion in his job by using to advantage the convalescent period.

It is evident when one appreciates the place which the thumb holds in the field of sensibility and in its cortical representation, that an operation such as pollicisation must involve a major alteration in the body pattern. Much effort at re-adaptation is involved. The latter is of such importance that should patients be adjudged incapable of actively participating in, and persevering with, their rehabilitation, they should be considered psychologically inadequate or should they show lack of will-power, then, in our opinion, they are not suitable for this operation.

14. RESULTS OF THUMB RECONSTRUCTION

F. Langlais and J. Gosset

The 45 pollicisations in our series were performed under two different sets of circumstances.

1. In 33 cases pollicisation was performed using a normal finger for an isolated lesion of the thumb. This we call a 'typical' pollicisation and we now use the ring finger for this procedure.

2. In the 12 other cases the hand had already sustained several lesions in addition to the trauma to the thumb. In these cases we restored thumb function by transferring a damaged index finger and we call this an 'atypical' pollicisation.

TYPICAL POLLICISATION FOR ISOLATED AMPUTATIONS OF THE THUMB

The majority of these patients (32 out of 33) had their operations at the St Antoine Hospital under the care of Professor Jean Gosset. There was only one pollicisation using a normal index at the Cochin Hospital where the use of an innervated tubed flap is standard in reconstruction of the isolated amputation of the thumb.

All the patients were followed-up for a minimum of 5 months. Twenty-one were reviewed from the point of view of function and occupation with an average follow-up of 3 years.

It should be noted that the majority of the patients had sustained a slicing type of injury and this is a favourable feature if reimplantation is to be undertaken by microsurgical technique.

WHY HAVE WE SUGGESTED POLLICISATION TO THE PATIENT?

It would perhaps seem illogical to sacrifice a normal finger (even if it is the ring finger which may not seem essential) to reconstruct the thumb. However, it appeared to us to be the technique offering the best chance of reproducing normal appearance and function of the thumb.

It does this in two ways. First of all by the strength and mobility of the new thumb, this mobility being due to the metacarpophalangeal and interphalangeal joints. This allows fine grip either pulp to pulp, or pulp to nail, and above all allows the use of tools by flexion of the fingers, holding the handle in the first web space. It is interesting to note the strength of the flexor tendons of the transposed finger compared with the thenar muscles themselves.

Secondly by the sensation, epicritic, stereognostic and above all proprioceptive which come automatically in this type of transposition.

The pollicisation therefore, is not a sacrifice of the ring finger but an improved use of it. The ring finger represents 10 per cent of the functional capacity of the hand, whereas the thumb represents some 40 per cent, so in sacrificing the ring finger to make a thumb there were gains in the region of 30 per cent.

WHICH FINGER SHOULD BE USED?

Of these 33 typical pollicisations, eight were performed using the index finger (used for the reason of proximity). On one occasion the middle finger was used and on 25 occasions the ring finger. We now use this as a standard procedure.

We will now list the reasons why we no longer use the other fingers.

The index finger. The index finger is most important in thumb/finger function, being used for pulp to pulp, pulp to nail, lateral and three point pinch. It is perfectly adapted for this, stable on the 2nd metacarpal and controlled by the 1st dorsal interosseous. To transfer this finger would cause disturbance of basic pinch grip that is already a well established pattern of activity and substitutes for it, a thumb opposing the middle finger which is not so well adapted to that function. The difference of length between the index finger and the thumb produces an excessive length of the flexor tendon which means the flexor of the index has to be anastomosed to the original thumb flexor which further complicates the operation.

The middle finger. This is important in three point pinch and therefore its loss is more important than that of the ring finger. More importantly amputation of the middle finger is cosmetically less acceptable as the second metacarpal is not very mobile and cannot fall over to close the space made by the amputation.

The little finger. This is usually too small to produce an efficient thumb and moreover it is a very useful digit in holding the handle of a tool in the palm of the hand.

Thus it seems to us that the ring finger is the ideal digit to transfer in a typical pollicisation.

(a) it has the greatest potential for improvement in function
(b) its site means that the cosmetic defect is minimal in that the 3rd and 5th metacarpals are easily approximated
(c) in transposition it moves around the circumference of a circle, the centre of which is the carpal tunnel, so that the length of the flexor tendon is undisturbed.

OPERATIVE TECHNIQUE

We only note here the general principles of the technique which has already been described (Gosset) but these are the principles which we consider influence a favourable result.

Group 1—cases in which the amputation was in the middle part of the 1st metacarpal (19 out of 25) and thus enabled one to attach the proximal phalanx of the ring finger to the stump of the 1st metacarpal, the digit being transposed on a pedicle consisting of skin, neurovascular bundles and flexor tendons.

(a) The palmar incision is in the line of the centre of the 4th metacarpal and is at right angles to an incision on the thenar eminence from the stump to the base of the palm. This should preferably be a curved incision, a straight incision having produced scar contracture and limitation of movement in three of our cases.

(b) The neurovascular pedicle of the ring finger is raised by isolating the digital arteries in the 3rd and 4th interspaces and tying the branches to the ulnar aspect of the middle finger and radial aspect of the little finger. The perineurium of the interosseous nerve is opened and one can then perform an interfasicular dissection of the nerve, isolating the components going to the ring finger. The medial and lateral muscles of the thenar eminence are separated to produce a bed for the transposed finger.

(c) The preparation of the tendons is essential. The vinculae connecting the tendon to the region of the metacarpal are cut and the tendon freed just to the point at which it emerges from the carpal tunnel (J. Michon). We have had four cases out of 14 where active flexion was less than perfect due to inadequate mobilisation of the flexor tendons. In the one case in which we felt secondary tenolysis was indicated the patient refused operation.

On the dorsum of the hand the extensor apparatus is cut, with particular emphasis on the expansion of the interosseous muscles because it is these that are used in the anastomosis to give extension of the new thumb rather than the extensor communis itself.

The ring finger is disarticulated at the metacarpophalangeal joint and moved towards the palm based on its skin and neurovascular pedicle.

(d) The ring finger is fixed to the 1st metacarpal either by a mortice joint or by Kirschner wires. It is necessary to rotate the transposed finger about 120° to ensure pulp to pulp opposition.

(e) The repair of the extensor apparatus is difficult but important. In the majority of the cases we have sutured the short extensor to the expansion of the ulnar interosseous and the long extensor to the expansion of the radial interosseous. In seven out of 14 cases the tension was wrong. Four cases had extension lag of about 20° at the proximal interphalangeal joint and three cases had a more severe extension lag at the level of the metacarpophalangeal joint.

Proximal amputations at the level of the base of the metacarpal (two cases) gave a much worse result than those at a more distal level in the metacarpal.

A proximal amputation, particularly at the level of the carpometacarpal joint is very difficult to manage with a tubed flap in that it lacks thenar muscles and the joint. This problem is more readily dealt with by pollicisation. The absence of the intrinsic muscles may be partially compensated by the action of the extrinsics. The flexor can produce at the same time a component of adduction if the pulleys are made fairly distally allowing them to act as a cord in the arc from the carpal tunnel to the distal phalanx. One of the extensor tendons of the thumb may be reinserted into the diaphysis of the proximal phalanx of the ring finger to produce abduc-

tion. Loss of the carpometacarpal joint can be made good by transferring the ring finger together with its metacarpophalangeal joint.

Results of two pollicisations for proximal amputations are the worst in our series. The first was a confectioner, aged 17, who had very poor extension of the new thumb. Despite this he carried on with his original job and did not want any further operation to shorten the extensors. The second was a labourer, aged 19, who had good movement but never used the transposed finger as a thumb. He also went back to his original occupation.

RESULTS OF TYPICAL POLLICISATION

There were no ischaemic complications and in all cases a good functional result was rapidly achieved.

We report 21 typical pollicisations with a follow-up of between 3 and 23 years.

(1) *Seven pollicisations using an index finger*. These are the first cases in our series (1947–1954). In this group there are some rather poor results corresponding to the time when the technique was still being modified. There are two bad results with poor mobility and a bad cosmetic appearance, three mediocre results and two good ones. They are graded out of a score of 10 depending on mobility, sensation and professional use and have an average score of 6·6. We no longer use this type of pollicisation.

(2) *Fourteen pollicisations of the ring finger*. In this group the average mark was 7·5 with nine very good results, three good and two average. The mobility was satisfactory in all cases and, we feel, was due to the degree of original flexor tendon mobilisation and the reinsertion of the extensors. In 11 cases function was comparable with that of a normal thumb with fine pinch, normal opposition, ability to open the first web space, good functional capacity in handling tools and the ability to carry more than 3 kg weight on the thumb.

It was sensation which ensured the return to previous occupation. Two-point discrimination was always good, usually in the region of 10 mm. There were no cases of pain at the donor site. Two-thirds of the patients complained of hypersensitivity to cold in the first year. Stereognostic sensation allowed the patient to appreciate the position of the new thumb without visualising it and this seems to be initiated by mechanoreceptors in thenar and extrinsic muscles. The stereognostic sensation when combined with epicritic sensation allows early overall integration of the thumb.

Proprioceptive sensation allows the patient to integrate the new thumb automatically. The thumb is initially considered as the transposed ring finger by the patient and then there is an intermediate phase which is unpleasant for the patient when sensation is related both to ring finger and thumb. There is finally complete integration which is probably dependent on mobility and the degree of recovery of sensation of the other two modalities.

Amongst 14 patients, 12 regarded the transposed digit as a normal thumb at between 3 months and 2 years. In two cases the finger was never recognised as a thumb and was only used when controlled by sight. In one of these the amputation was proximal to the carpometacarpal joint, in the other there was a neuroma. Functional recovery was good in all 21 pollicisations, for the most part in manual workers, despite the variety of techniques we used.

In 18 manual workers, 16 had returned to exactly the same job on average 4 months after the pollicisation, the needs of strength and/or precision being well represented in the group. Two manual workers did not get back to their original occupation: a confectioner, aged 19, was never able to integrate his ring finger and now works in a chemical laboratory. A cabinet maker, aged 63, has retired despite a good result. In the non-manual workers, function was rapidly re-achieved. A child of eight soon went back to school and a director of a firm was back in his office within 20 days. A patient, aged 64, who had an amputation for a carcinoma of the thumb was already an invalid before the pollicisation.

The rapid return to function we feel is a result of performing the whole reconstruction in one operation and only infrequently was it necessary to re-operate to adjust the length of the tendons.

In our experience pollicisation of the ring finger offers the best method of reconstructing the thumb for the following reasons:

(i) It is one operation, with a low complication rate and is a less complicated procedure than a tubed neurovascular flap and bone graft.
(ii) It produces a new thumb which is automatically used and can be used for fine manipulation or for handling tools.
(iii) It allows a manual worker to return to his original work with a delay in the region of six months.

ATYPICAL POLLICISATION FOR COMBINED LESIONS OF THE THUMB AND FINGERS

These are very different problems from those already discussed in that the amputation of a thumb is not the main element of the often considerable trauma to the hand. Amongst the 12 cases we report, 10 were the result of crushing or severe wounds and there were only two that could feasibly have been repaired by microsurgery.

In this sort of problem we cannot risk transferring a normal finger because of the danger of further decreasing the function of the mutilated hand. The goal of atypical pollicisation is simply to produce some improvement of thumb function by using a finger that has already been damaged, the loss of which will not reduce the overall function of the hand. In practice in our experience the index finger is the only one that can be transferred under these circumstances. If it is of full length but stiff it will interfere with grip between the new thumb and the middle finger and if it is mobile but short it cannot be opposed as a new thumb. It is the only finger that can be transferred without considerable operative risk in that it can be taken en masse with digital arteries based on the interosseous artery and the dorsal veins. Use of the index finger will allow the first web space to be considerably deepened.

In the 12 cases we are reporting, five of them were operated on at the Saint Antoine Hospital and seven at the Cochin Hospital. Details of operative technique were comparable. The index was taken as an island on a neurovascular pedicle without a skin flap. The relative lengths of the index and thumb stumps dictate the level of section taking the index either at the proximal phalanx or the metacarpal. Rotation of the new thumb and re-attachment of the extensor tendons are the same as for a typical pollicisation but the flexor tendon has to be anastomosed to that of the original thumb due to inequality of length.

CLINICAL RESULTS

The overall results were mediocre and do not compare with those achieved by transposing a normal finger.

1. Six cases showed no improvement at all. In two cases the levels of amputation in both the thumb and the index were too proximal. In one case we achieved a thumb which only reached the level of the distal palmar crease and was only used for opposition against a slightly stiff middle finger. In the other the amputation was at the level of the trapezium and produced a fixed adducted thumb despite using a trapezio-metacarpal replacement and a hypothenar muscle flap (Littler) to reproduce adduction plus an abductor tendon transfer. We therefore no longer consider pollicisation if the length of the thumb will not allow effective pinch against the middle finger or if all the musculature of the first ray has been destroyed.

In two cases there were ischaemic problems with the transferred index. One of these cases constitutes the only case in which necrosis necessitated an amputation. This was in a shotgun wound of the hand which obviously compromised the digital circulation. In the other, although viable, there was sepsis and subsequent stiffness.

In two cases an abdominal flap had already been used for partial loss of substance. There were trophic changes and the new thumb was of little use.

2. There were three mediocre results (score 4 out of 10) but even that represents considerable functional improvement in a severely mutilated hand. One of these results was achieved in a patient with an amputation of the thumb, loss of substance at the carpometacarpal level and a large wound of the medial forearm, where nerve suture was performed and the carpus arthrodesed.

3. There were three reasonable results (score 6 out of 10). These were in cases of amputation of the ulnar two digits with use of a slightly shortened or stiff index for the thumb.

Return to previous occupation is rare in these cases and only occurred in one out of five manual workers. He returned to printing but the other patients all required retraining.

These poor results contrast with the consistently good results of transfer of the normal ring finger. Improvement has only occurred in a small proportion of cases in the former group.

These results are too poor for us to recommend pollicisation in severe multilations and we now look to the microsurgeons to improve the prognosis in these cases.

15. THUMB RECONSTRUCTION IN THE MUTILATED HAND WITH SPECIAL REFERENCE TO POLLICISATION

D. A. Campbell Reid

Our experience of pollicisation as a means of thumb reconstruction is based on a personal series of 38 cases of which 20 were undertaken for congenital deficiency. This leaves 18 cases of traumatic thumb loss treated by this method and upon which our observations in this chapter are based. Inevitably, when discussing thumb reconstruction one must refer to the other main methods which are used, viz. the Gillies' thumb-stall lengthening procedure and reconstruction by tubed flap, bone graft and neurovascular island flap.

CLASSIFICATION OF THUMB LOSS

We use the classification which we originally described (Reid, 1960). This is based on the level of loss which we consider the main factor influencing the choice of treatment:

Group 1: Amputation distal to the metacarpophalangeal joint, leaving an adequate stump

Group 2: Amputation of the thumb distal to or through the metacarpophalgeal joint leaving a stump of inadequate length

Group 3: Amputation through the metacarpal with preservation of some functioning thenar muscles

Group 4: Amputation at or near the carpometacarpal joint with loss of all thenar muscles.

SELECTION OF CASES

It is not an easy decision for the patient to make when confronted with the possibility of reconstructive surgery after loss of a thumb. The various possibilities should be put to him as clearly and simply as possible, stressing the undoubted gain that is likely to be achieved. It is right to be confident and enthusiastic when suggesting pollicisation following major thumb loss but the decision must be left to the patient who should be given time to deliberate, having been given all the facts. It is not surprising that a number of patients will refuse reconstruction for various reasons. Some feel they can manage with the hand as it is and there is no doubt that others will turn down surgery as they consider they will get less compensation for their injury. Age, of course, is another factor and as a general rule we would not undertake major reconstruction over the age of 50 years.

We have never felt justified in undertaking pollicisation in group 2 cases where there has been an isolated loss of thumb with four intact fully functional fingers. It has been our experience that adequate thumb lengthening may be achieved in these cases either by a Gillies' thumb-stall lengthening

procedure or by the other osteoplastic procedure, namely bone graft, tubed pedicle and neurovascular island flap. Moreover, both these procedures in our hands, have given satisfactory results. The former method, in a one-stage operative procedure, gives a strong, stable thumb with sensation, the amount of lengthening being about 2·5 cm. This is perfectly adequate for satisfactory opposition to normal fingers and the aesthetic result is acceptable to a working man (Fig. 15.1). We have found, moreover, that early use of the reconstructed thumb seems to encourage consolidation of the bone graft. This is perfectly safe provided the following technique is used for inserting the graft. A 5 cm long full-thickness segment is taken from the iliac crest. The proximal 2·5 cm of this is prepared as a peg utilising the cortical bone. This preparation is readily achieved by using power-driven burrs. The metacarpal is reamed out to receive the peg which is then securely inserted for its full length. No other fixation is required.

The alternative method of thumb reconstruction in these cases is by bone graft, tubed pedicle and neurovascular island flap. It also gives satisfactory results and may be undertaken in two stages. The first necessitates the raising of a tubed flap, preferably a groin flap, the dimensions of which should be 7·5 cm wide by 10 cm in length. The base of the flap is also back-cut so that when tubed the seam will lie along the ulnar aspect. A bone graft is then taken from the iliac crest through the same incision, fashioned and pegged into the metacarpal as previously described. The projecting bone graft is now inserted into the tubed flap. The second stage is carried out 3 weeks later. The tubed flap is divided and a neurovascular island flap taken from the ulnar aspect of the ring or middle finger is let into the seam and closes the end of the tube. A typical result of such a procedure is shown in figure 15.2. This was in a young woman of 18 years, and with an artificial nail added to the thumb, the latter is not unattractive. This patient has been followed up for 6 years and has excellent function.

Loss of thumb associated with mutilations of one or more digits, in our opinion, is the ideal indication for pollicisation using a mutilated digit, provided that digit has normal sensation. The principle of combining two deficient digits in this way to make one effective functioning one, a thumb, is a sound one. A high proportion of our cases, 14 out of 18 had associated injury to other digits (Table 15.1). The distribution of cases according to grouping is shown in table 15.2. The digit pollicised in cases of multiple mutilations is indicated in table 15.3. It will be seen that most of these were group 2 cases. The main object in these cases is to lengthen the thumb sufficiently for pinch and grasp. The outlook is good since the all-important carpometacarpal joint is functional. There was only one group 3 case. Here the sole remaining undamaged finger was the little one. It was not considered justifiable to pollicise this and the index metacarpal with normal sensibility in its overlying skin was used. Of the four cases of isolated thumb loss with four intact fingers, two were group 3 cases and two group 4. It was considered entirely justifiable to pollicise an intact normal finger in group 3 cases and one may anticipate excellent results in such cases since opposition and abduction are present.

POLLICISATION IN GROUP 2 CASES

There were eight cases in this group and in each case loss of the thumb in the region of the metacarpophalangeal joint was associated with loss of the index and/or middle, ring and little fingers through the proximal phalanges or metacarpophalangeal joints. The index stump was pollicised in seven cases. The technique was that described by Littler (1953), i.e. radial migration of the index stump on its neurovascular pedicles. The technique is illustrated in figure 15.3. The

TABLE 15.1

18 CASES	
ISOLATED LOSS OF THUMB	ASSOCIATED INJURY TO OTHER DIGITS
4	14

Figure 15.1
A, Preoperative view of case presenting with loss of thumb just distal to metacarpophalangeal joint.
B, Thumb lengthening 10 days after operation.
C, End result showing strong, stable thumb. Note the bone graft, with peg into metacarpal, becoming well incorporated.

A   B

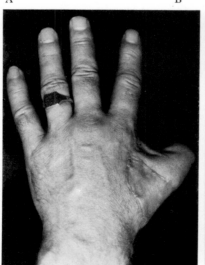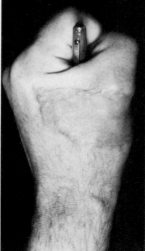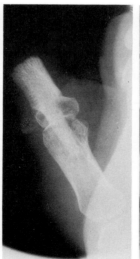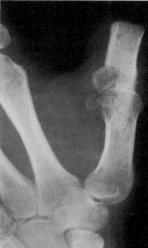

C

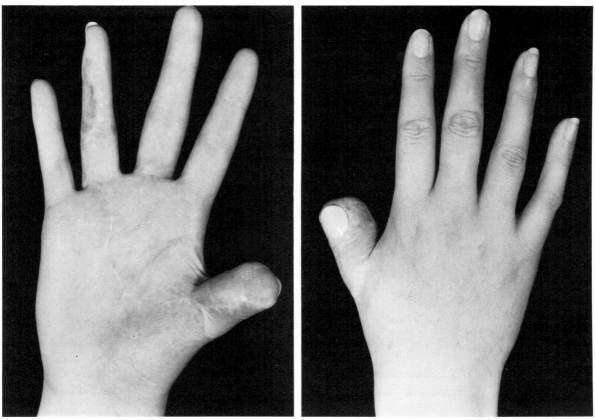

Figure 15.2
Result of thumb reconstruction by tubed pedicle, bone graft and island flap. Note that the island flap covers the whole of the tactile surface of the thumb, the tubed flap having been reduced by excision over the dorsum. An artificial nail has been attached.

incisions are first marked out, a flap is outlined on the dorsum of the thumb/index web and based on its palmar aspect. The base of the index stump is then circumscribed at the level of the metacarpophalangeal joint and the racket type incision completed by a tongue-like extension on the dorsum of the hand. The flaps are raised and the web flap reflected back so as to expose the palmar aspect. The digital nerve to the radial side of the index and the radialis indicis artery are exposed and carefully dissected back into the palm. The neurovascular bundle to the index/middle cleft is then exposed by dividing the palmar aponeurosis and this is also dissected back into the

palm. The division of the common volar digital artery is exposed and the branch to the radial side of the middle finger divided and ligated well clear of the bifurcation. The corresponding nerves to the adjacent sides of the cleft are readily separated by fine scissor dissection as far back as is necessary. The flexor tendons are not disturbed in the dissection. The structures in the 2nd/3rd intermetacarpal space are now divided starting on the dorsum whilst keeping careful watch on the vessels and nerves already displayed in the palm. The deep transverse intermetacarpal ligament is divided and then the interossei in the cleft are separated from one another by

TABLE 15.2

GROUPS			
I	II	III	IV
0	8	1	5

TABLE 15.3

MUTILATED DIGIT USED FOR POLLICISATION			
INDEX	MIDDLE	RING	LITTLE
9	3	1	1

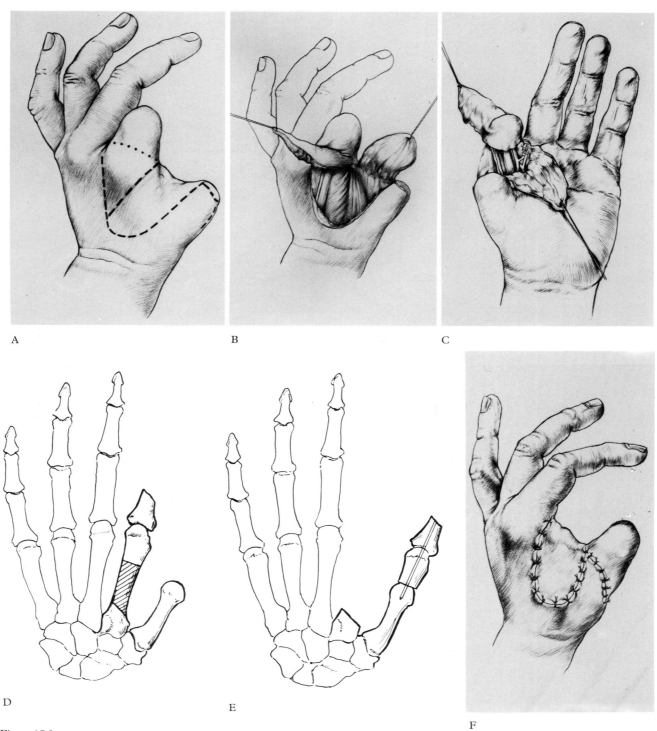

A

B

C

D

E

F

Figure 15.3
A, Flaps outlined.
B, Flaps raised.
C, Neurovascular bundles displayed in palm. Digital artery to radial side of middle finger ligated.
D, The part of the 2nd metacarpal to be discarded is cross-hatched.
E, Fixation of pollicised index stump.
F, Skin closure is illustrated.

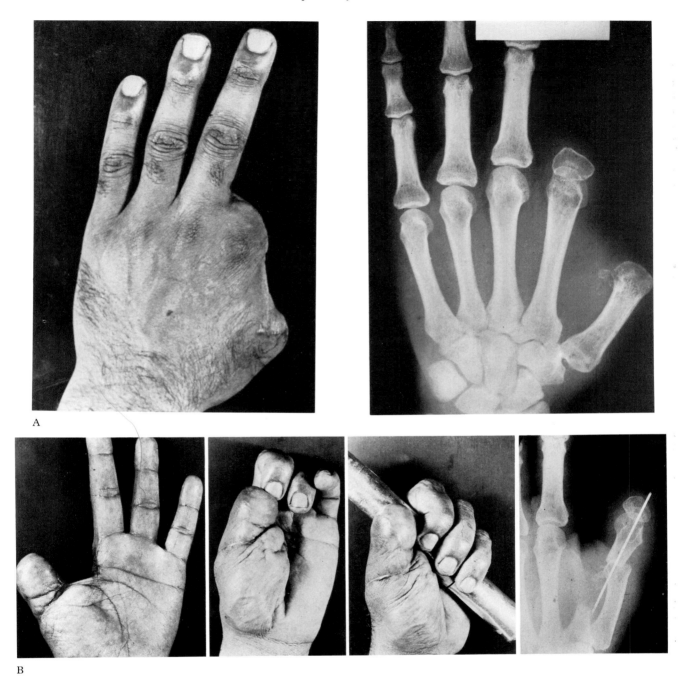

Figure 15.4
A, Condition of left hand prior to reconstruction. Note the rather short index stump.
B, Result of pollicisation of index stump.

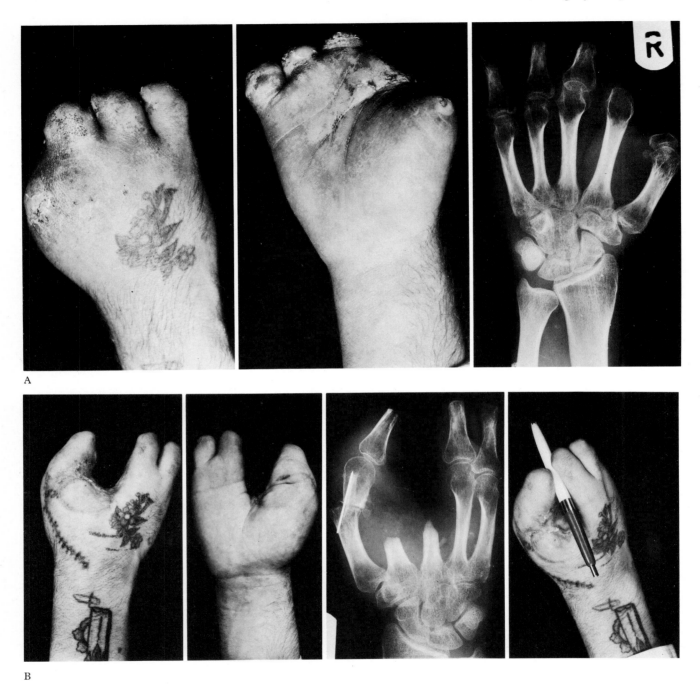

A

B

Figure 15.5
A, Initial condition, the result of a circular saw injury, prior to reconstruction. Note short index stump on X-ray, unsuitable for pollicisation.
B, Result of pollicisation of middle finger stump. Note that the index metacarpal has been removed.

blunt dissection well back to the proximal part of the space. The extensor tendons are left undisturbed.

Final mobilisation of the digit requires division of the index metacarpal. This is exposed sub-periosteally near its base and along its radial side. The extensor tendons are displaced in an ulnar direction. The metacarpal is divided obliquely near its base using an oscillating saw. The metacarpal is recessed, removing a segment by a second, more distally placed, saw cut, transverse this time and at such a level as to allow comfortable transfer of the digit. The main factor controlling this is the length of the neurovascular bundles which must not be embarrassed by any degree of tension. The index stump will now be entirely mobile, its only remaining attachments being its two neurovascular pedicles and its flexor and extensor tendons.

The thumb stump is now prepared by freshening its end to expose raw bone. The index stump is then transposed so that its metacarpal sits on the thumb metacarpal. Fixation is achieved by one or two Kirschner wires which are cut short and buried beneath the skin. The tourniquet is now released and bleeding controlled. Skin closure is effected by transposing the web flap to fill the defect.

Pollicisation in a typical group 2 case is shown in figure 15.4. The patient presented for reconstruction following a mutilating injury in which left thumb and index finger had been amputated by an axe. The thumb was lost through the metacarpophalangeal joint and the index finger just beyond the joint. Excellent function was obtained in this one-stage operative procedure. It was necessary to apply split skin grafts to the sides of the new thumb/middle finger cleft but the web itself was covered with the dorsal flap. This was the result of the rather short index stump. The new thumb was, however, sufficiently long to oppose to the middle and ring fingers.

A severely mutilated hand (phalangeal hand), the result of a circular saw accident is shown in figure 15.5. In this case the index metacarpal was too short for useful pollicisation. It was therefore removed and the middle finger used instead. This possessed an effective metacarpophalangeal joint. In the transfer, flexor tendons were taken and the extensor digitorum tendon was divided and linked to the extensor pollicis longus at wrist level. Part of the adductor pollicis attachment was left on the remaining part of the 3rd metacarpal. Satisfactory function with a useful grasp mechanism resulted. In another severe mutilation, also a circular saw injury, thumb, index, middle and ring fingers were amputated at metacarpophalangeal joint level, only the little finger surviving unscathed. The index metacarpal was pollicised giving a rather short thumb which failed to oppose to the little finger (Fig. 15.6). This was readily remedied by performing a rotation osteotomy on the 5th metacarpal. He now has excellent opposition and grasping function.

RESULTS IN GROUP 2 CASES

The functional results in six of the eight cases were satisfactory fulfilling the requirements of a reconstructed thumb (Tanzer and Littler, 1948). Five of these were excellent

G

results whilst the other one was only marred by a somewhat reduced web space due to excessive scarring. This could readily be rectified by further grafting. The two remaining cases could only be classified as fair results. In one of them, there had been damage at the time of injury to the 1st inter-metacarpal space. Nevertheless a grasping mechanism was obtained. In the other, although a grasp was obtained the pollicised digit remained in a somewhat too flexed position. The cases in this group had been undertaken from 1 to 20 years previously, seven of them over 5 years before.

POLLICISATION IN GROUP 3 CASES

We have again used the Littler technique in these reconstructions. In two cases we pollicised an intact undamaged index finger whilst in the third, a badly mutilated hand, only the little finger remained undamaged and we used the index stump. This left rather a short thumb and it was subsequently necessary to perform rotation osteotomies of the 3rd, 4th and 5th metacarpals. This resulted in a useful grasping hand, the little finger being of most value.

The technique is illustrated in figure 15.7. The incisions used were those described by Littler (1953) although a modification of this described by Barsky (1965) is a good alternative and one we have employed for most of our reconstructions for congenital absence or hypoplasia of the thumb. Here the incision is in the form of an S on the radial side of the hand providing two flaps, the more distal one based on the palmar aspect and the more proximal on the dorsal aspect. In traumatic cases, the design of the flaps may have to be modified depending on the site of scarring. The initial steps of the operation are exactly as described for group 2 cases. The index finger is recessed by removal of most of its metacarpal and the base of the proximal phalanx. Flexor and extensor tendons are transferred intact with minimum disturbance. The pollicised digit is fixed in the optimal position of rotation on the thumb metacarpal, and we have found that the most certain way of achieving this is by the use of an intramedullary bone graft transfixed by two Kirschner wires passed transversely. The operation is completed by suturing the web flap into the new web.

We have found that the slack in both flexor and extensor tendons is taken up spontaneously within a few months and secondary tendon adjustments are rarely required. A stable lad had the unusual misfortune to have his thumb bitten off by a racehorse he was attending. The result of pollicisation is shown in figure 15.8.

RESULTS IN GROUP 3 CASES

The fact that the carpometacarpal joint is intact and has sufficient surviving thenar muscles to activate it ensures a satisfactory outcome in this group. In both cases where we were able to pollicise an intact index finger, the results both functionally and aesthetically were entirely satisfactory.

In the third case, as already described, a useful hand was obtained after pollicisation of the index metacarpal followed by rotation osteotomies of the other digits.

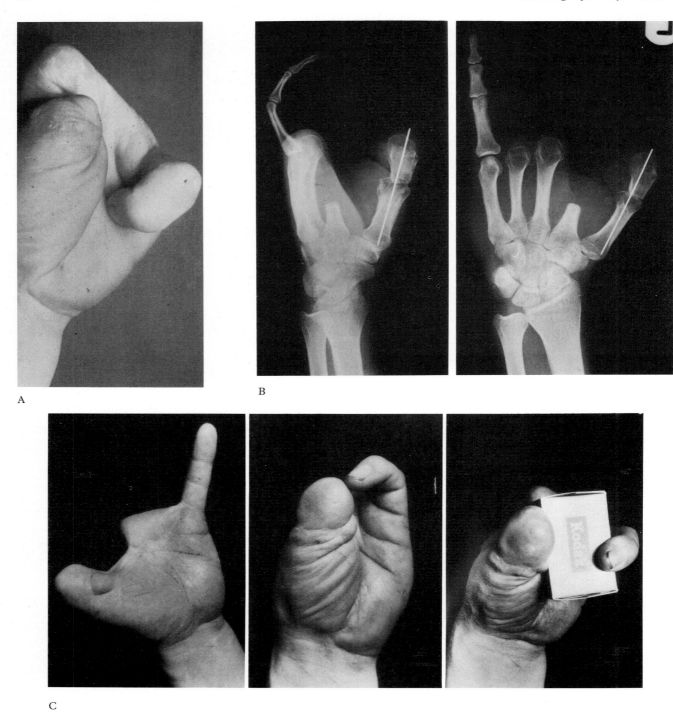

Figure 15.6
A, Hand prior to reconstruction. The little finger failed to meet the thumb stump.
B, X-ray appearance following pollicisation of the index metacarpal.
C, Final result following rotation osteotomy through the 5th metacarpal. Note the satisfactory opposition and grasp.

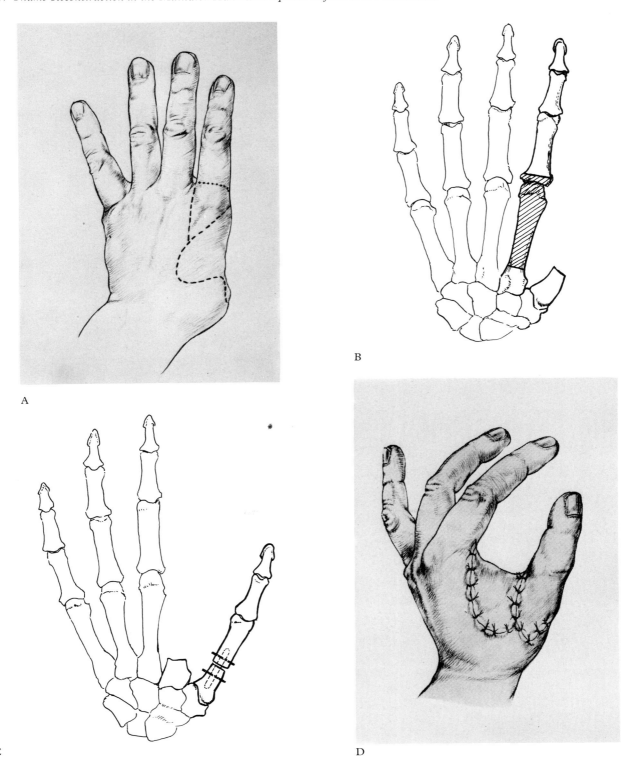

Figure 15.7
A, Outline of incisions.
B, The amount of bone to be resected is cross-hatched.
C, Technique for fixation of pollicised digit using intramedullary bone graft and cross K wires.
D, Pollicisation completed.

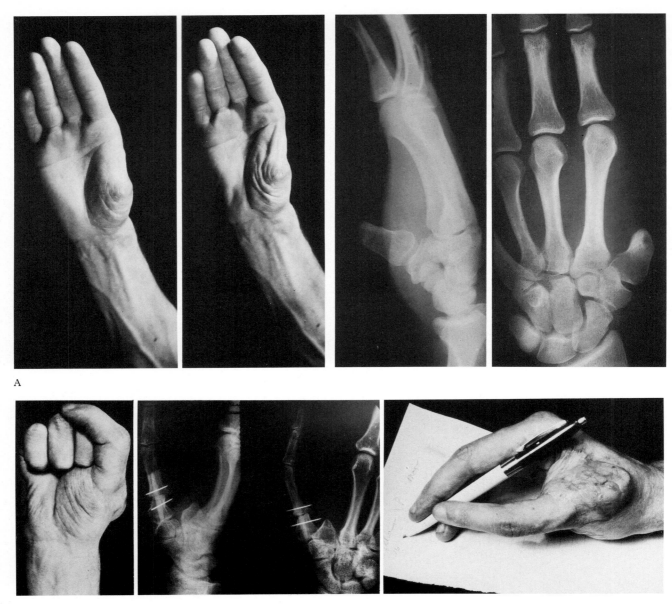

A

B

Figure 15.8
A, Hand prior to pollicisation. Note the short though mobile stump of 1st metacarpal.
B, Result of pollicisation. X-rays show fixation of intramedullary bone graft.

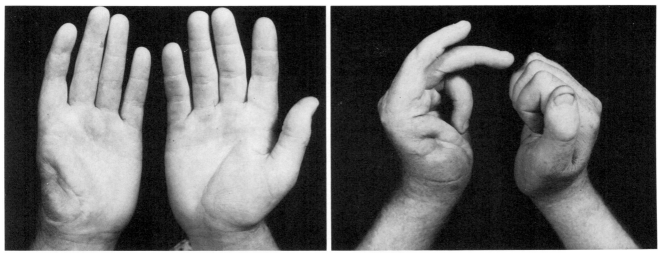

A

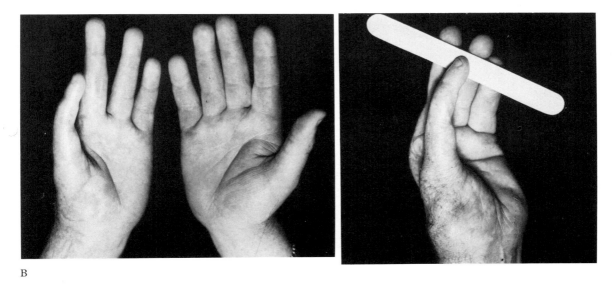

B

Figure 15.9
A, Total amputation of left thumb in circular saw accident. The proximal interphalangeal joints of index and middle fingers were also damaged resulting in gross limitation of flexion of these fingers.
B, Result of pollicisation of stiff index finger including the mobile metacarpophalangeal joint. Note the new thumb though ungainly in appearance has a useful pinch grip with the stiff middle finger.

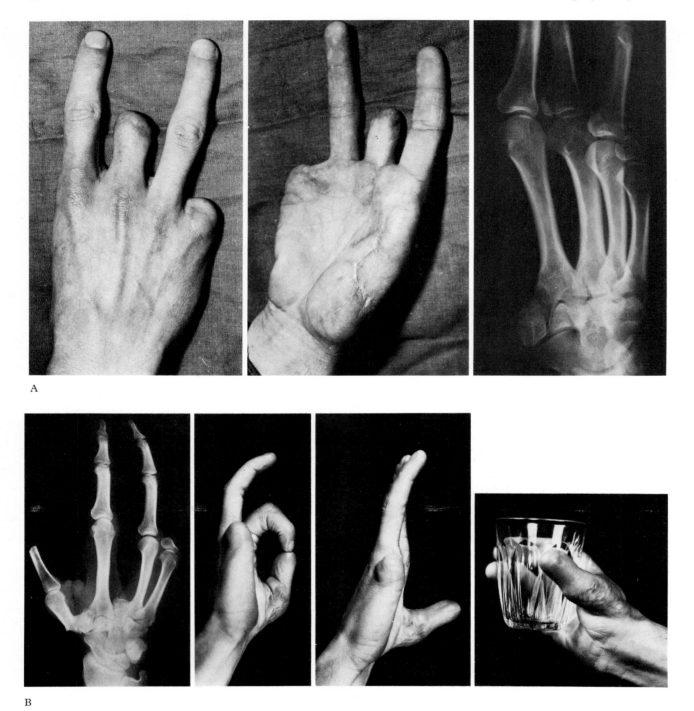

Figure 15.10
A, Initial condition of the hand presenting for reconstruction. X-ray shows total loss of 1st metacarpal.
B, Functional result following pollicisation of the middle finger stump. Note the excellent pinch and also grasp for larger objects. X-ray shows sound fusion of the pollicised digit with the trapezium.

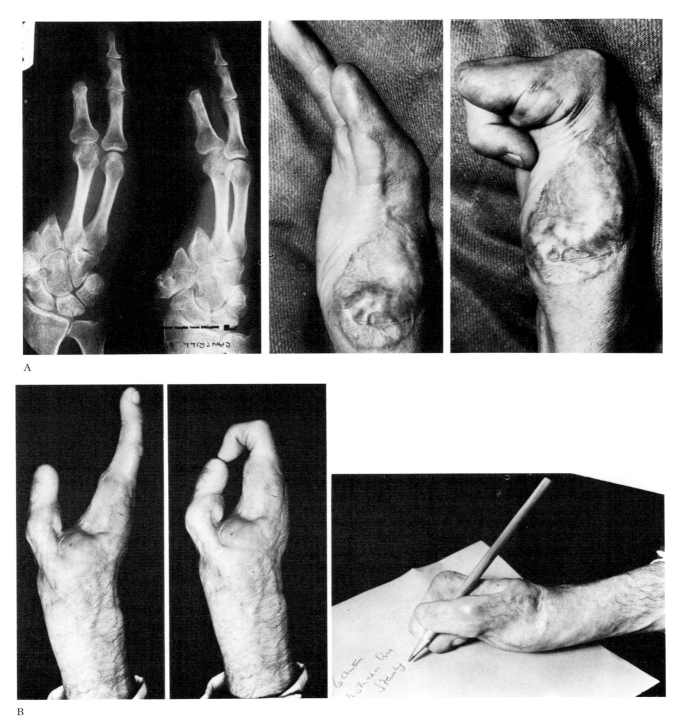

Figure 15.11
A, Severe radial hemiamputation of the hand prior to reconstruction.
B, Result following pollicisation of ring finger stump in one operation.

POLLICISATION IN GROUP 4 INJURIES

There were seven cases in this group, five with multiple digit injury and two only with isolated loss of the thumb.

In the five multiple digit injuries, the index finger was pollicised in one case, the middle in two, the ring in one and the little finger in one. In the other group the index finger was pollicised in both instances. The technique of pollicisation was varied according to circumstances in each particular case. Where the index finger was pollicised this was by the usual radial migration neurovascular pedicle method. In two of our early cases where pollicisation of an index finger was undertaken for an isolated loss of thumb, we did not include the metacarpophalangeal joint as we felt that its inclusion would provide too long a thumb. Whilst the results were satisfactory, we feel that the metacarpophalangeal joint should be preserved with as short a segment of metacarpal neck as possible, this being attached to the trapezium if present or, failing that, the base of the 2nd metacarpal. In one case, as a result of a circular saw accident the patient, in addition to losing his thumb, was left with stiff interphalangeal joints of index and middle fingers (Fig. 15.9). Pollicisation of the index finger here included a slightly longer length of metacarpal than usual. Although the new thumb is too long and looks ugly, it provides the necessary movement and opposes satisfactorily against the stiff middle finger.

The middle finger stump was pollicised by a modified Hilgenfeldt technique. This was a circular saw injury with total loss of thumb associated with loss of middle finger at proximal interphalangeal joint level and little finger at metacarpophalangeal joint level. Index and ring fingers were undamaged (Fig. 15.10). The metacarpophalangeal joint was included in the transfer with removal of the proximal part of the 3rd metacarpal. The flexor tendons were also transferred. The extensor tendon was divided well back in the hand and linked to extensor pollicis longus at wrist level. The pollicised digit was transposed by tunnelling it through to the radial side of the hand deep to the skin bridge between the palmar incision and a web flap on the radial side. The metacarpal was then fixed to the trapezium after removing its articular surface. Two Kirschner wires ensured sound union. The secondary defect on the dorsum of the hand left by raising a large web flap was covered with a split-skin graft.

In the other case where the middle finger stump was utilised, both 1st and 2nd rays had also been lost. In addition, the neurovascular bundle to the radial side of the middle finger stump had been divided. In spite of this, pollicisation was accomplished by radial migration of the stump, with no problems and the opposable surface of the new thumb had sensation.

The ring finger stump was pollicised in another severe radial hemiamputation (Fig. 15.11). The patient, a man aged 31, had sustained the injury to his right hand by a circular saw 7 months previously. A one-stage pollicisation of the ring finger stump, including most of its metacarpal was undertaken. Flexor and extensor tendons were transferred with the digit which was implanted on the radial side of the carpus and

the cleft lined with split-skin grafts. An excellent functional result was achieved. This reconstruction brought about a most dramatic psychological change in the patient's outlook. Whereas, before the operation he was morose and introspective, always keeping the mutilated hand out of sight in his pocket, once he had a hand which he could use, he became cheerful and industrious and lost all self-consciousness of his mutilated hand. He returned to work and, in fact, soon assumed a position of increased responsibility.

The fifth of the multiple injuries in this group was a patient who again had sustained radial hemiamputation with total loss of 1st and 2nd rays. The vascularity of the middle finger was suspect and it was decided to pollicise the little finger. Much scarring was encountered in the palm of the hand and after transfer the little finger remained congested postoperatively. Intravenous low molecular weight dextran was started at once and continued for 4 days and the pollicised digit recovered completely. Sensation, deficient initially, also recovered. The result in this case has been an indifferent one although a pinch has been provided between the digit and the other two fingers.

RESULTS IN GROUP 4 CASES

Of the five multiple digit injuries there were two excellent results, transfers of middle and ring stumps with fully mobile metacarpophalangeal joints. Transfer of an index finger with stiff proximal interphalangeal joint but including the metacarpophalangeal joint achieved a good functional result opposing well to a stiff middle finger. The other case where a middle finger stump was used and transferred on the remaining neurovascular pedicle was a reasonable result though there was some limitation of spread of the new thumb. The little finger pollicisation as already stated was only a fair result.

SUMMARY

Experience of pollicisation in 18 cases of traumatic thumb loss is described. Our routine is to use an alternative method of reconstruction for thumb loss at metacarpophalangeal joint level when all four fingers are undamaged. The majority of cases had mutilated digits which could be usefully pollicised. The technique of pollicisation and the results are described in group 2, 3 and 4 cases.

BIBLIOGRAPHY

Barsky, A. J. (1965). Migration of a radial digit on a neurovascular pedicle. In *The Proceedings of The Second Hand Club*, p. 314. Published by the British Society for Surgery of the Hand, 1975.

Littler, J. W. (1953). Neurovascular pedicle method of digital transposition for reconstruction of the thumb. *Plastic and Reconstructive Surgery*, **12,** 303.

Reid, D. A. Campbell (1960). Reconstruction of the thumb. *Journal of Bone and Joint Surgery*, **42B,** 648.

Reid, D. A. Campbell (1969). Pollicisation—an appraisal. *The Hand*, **1,** 27.

Tanzer, R. C. & Littler, J. W. (1948). Reconstruction of the thumb. *Plastic and Reconstructive Surgery*, **3,** 533.

16. RECONSTRUCTION OF THE THUMB BY TUBE PEDICLE, BONE GRAFT AND ISLAND FLAP

C. Simonetta

In 1900, Nicoladoni described a reconstruction of the thumb by tube pedicle and bone graft since when, this method remained without major modifications until recently. Thumbs reconstructed in this way were not really satisfactory owing to their excessive bulk of soft tissue, their tendency to skin instability at the tip and their poor sensibility. Moreover, complications such as trophic ulcers and bone resorption were not infrequent.

The transfer of an island flap based on a neurovascular bundle was suggested by Moberg in 1955 and first put into practice by Littler in 1956. The main application of this brilliant technique was, of course, the reconstructed thumb as it enabled one to bring to the tip nearly normal sensation and an excellent blood supply.

In order to reduce the chance of bone resorption, we introduced a composite bone–skin flap (McGregor and Simonetta, 1961). This soon proved to be an unnecessary precaution as the island flap, brought through at the time the tube was divided and placed in close contact with the bone, introduced an adequate blood supply. A free bone graft was easier to shape properly and to fix in the right position.

The reconstructed thumb, however, still presented several defects:

1. The sensitive skin brought with the island flap was limited as only the hemipulp distal to the terminal interphalangeal joint was taken from the ring finger and its width was no more than 1 cm
2. This island flap was too often excessively mobile on its bony support and this reduced pinch precision and stability
3. Raising a flap from the deltopectoral region created an unsightly scar in an exposed area.

We think that these problems have been solved with some improvements and modifications of technique.

PRINCIPLE OF THE METHOD

A groin flap (Fig. 16.1) as described by McGregor (McGregor and Jackson, 1971) and including the superficial circumflex iliac artery, is raised on the same side as the hand whose thumb is to be reconstructed (Fig. 16.2). This flap must have a width of 7·5 cm and a minimum length of 12·0 cm, its free end being on the top of the iliac crest. The bone graft (Fig. 16.3) is taken from the crest and one has to be careful to shape it as a racket 7 to 8 mm thick, 5 to 6 cm long and 1·5 cm wide. This shape will limit the risk of skin movement around the bone. The bone graft is then introduced

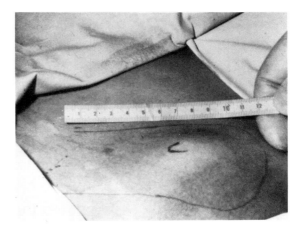

Figure 16.1
Drawing of the groin flap which is 12 cm long and 7 cm wide.

into the 1st metacarpal shaft and orientated so that its flat aspect is facing the index finger in opposition. Fixation is secured by a screw or pins. The groin flap is tubed along most of its length after a partial defatting, which is not always necessary since the subcutaneous fat forms quite a thin layer in this area (Fig. 16.4). The groin crease is closed by direct suture without excessive tension, no free skin graft being necessary. The bone graft is inserted inside the tube, the suture line of which is placed on the volar aspect, where the island flap will be sited at a subsequent stage. The free end of

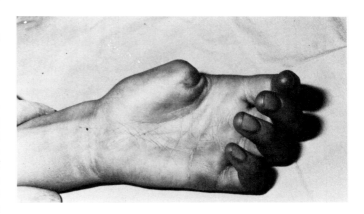

Figure 16.2
Amputation of the thumb at the metacarpophalangeal joint.

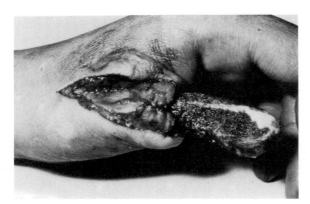

Figure 16.3
The bone peg shaped as a racket, is inserted into the metacarpal.

the tube pedicle is sutured to a large oval area extending on to the dorsum almost as far as the base of the 1st metacarpal. This will encourage numerous vascular connections with the recipient stump. The position of the upper limb is a comfortable and natural one so that immobilisation with strapping is only required for a few days. The patient may be discharged from hospital after about a week.

The excellent blood supply of the groin flap has the disadvantage that it does not adequately stimulate the circulation coming from the hand. A partial division of the flap has to be carried out after 4 weeks. Under local anaesthesia a transverse incision is made at the level of the future division of the tube and the superficial circumflex iliac artery is isolated and ligated. Six weeks after the first operation, the division of the tube is completed. An island flap (Fig. 16.5) is raised on the middle or ring finger. It must be of sufficient length, e.g. as far proximally as the proximal interphalangeal joint and about 2 cm wide. For this it must extend on to the dorsal aspect of the finger. A partial excision of the volar part of the tube allows one to place the island flap exactly on top of the flat surface of the bone graft and to close the open end of the tube (Fig. 16.6).

Thumb reconstruction is then completed in 6 weeks after only two main operations. The residual scar in the groin may be covered by even the smallest bikini.

INDICATIONS

Many factors such as age, sex, profession and co-operation, must be considered before deciding whether a patient would benefit from thumb reconstruction. The method will depend on the level of amputation and on whether there are associated amputations in the other digits.

RESULTS

A review of our statistics revealed that undoubtedly the best functional and cosmetic results have been obtained in reconstructions for subtotal amputations of the thumb. These

are cases where the thumb has been amputated between the proximal third of the proximal phalanx and the distal third of the metacarpal. They have in common, an intact carpometacarpal joint and functioning thenar muscles but the stump is too short to provide a fine pinch and a good grip. In this group, the length of the new thumb corresponds to a thumb which has lost its distal phalanx, and it is well known how readily patients can adapt themselves to such a mutilation. Fine pinch and grasp are possible and only the absence of the nail limits the capacity for very precise work. Cosmetically, the reconstructed thumb has a calibre which approximates more to that of a normal thumb than does a pollicised digit. In spite of the absence of the metacarpophalangeal joint, the mobile carpometacarpal joint and the intact thenar muscles make possible all the essential movements.

Reconstruction of the thumb following total amputation led to much inferior results from both functional and cosmetic points of view. We include in this group amputations between the middle of the metacarpal and the carpometacarpal joint, and in all these cases, the function of the carpometacarpal joint was very limited or absent. The situation is virtually the same as in congenital absence, and reconstruction by tube pedicle and bone graft will give a poor-looking short and stiff stump. Pollicisation of the index finger, however, is the only procedure which can bring intrinsic muscles to replace the thenar ones and a metacarpophalangeal joint which can act as a carpometacarpal one.

Total amputation of the thumb is very often associated with more or less severe damage to other digits and especially of the index finger. If an intact finger cannot be spared to be pollicised, transposition of a finger stump must be contemplated but if the finger remnants cannot be spared, reconstruction with tube pedicle and bone graft may be the only possible method available. To quote an example, we have reconstructed both thumbs of a postman who lost the thumb in addition to the index and middle fingers of both hands, in an explosion. No thenar muscles were left. We inserted bone

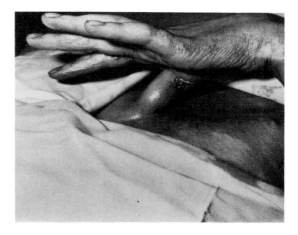

Figure 16.4
The tubed groin flap in place.

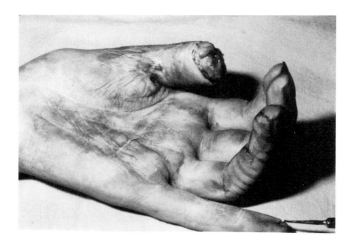

Figure 16.5
Raising of the island flap at time of division of the tube pedicle.

grafts directly into each trapezium. In spite of the rigidity and shortness of these thumbs, the patient was able to resume normal work handling hundreds of letters and parcels every day. In several other cases of thumb amputation at the same level, the rudimentary stump created with a tube pedicle and bone graft has proved to be a very useful procedure provided the skin over the end of the bone has been stable and possessed of normal sensation.

Instability of the skin over the bone graft was a common finding when fat abdominal tubes were used. This may be avoided by carefully tightening the partially defatted groin tube around the island flap which should then lie immediately over the flat surface of the bone graft.

Sometimes, a final correction may be necessary several months after reconstruction has been completed, because the island flap has spread in the meantime. After excising excess of the tube, the island flap is further spread and will be found to cover a much bigger area than originally and this will improve the quality of pinch and grasp.

ESTIMATION OF DISABILITY

It has been claimed by Littler that pollicisation is a highly beneficial operation as it results in a strategic revaluation of the transposed digit. This would be true if the pollicised digit gave a normal looking and functioning thumb but this is never the case.

In a subtotal amputation, pollicisation of the ring finger (worth 10 per cent) will give, in the best cases, a thumb worth 30 per cent (40 per cent is the value of a normal thumb). Reconstruction by tube pedicle and bone graft gives a thumb worth 20 per cent at least. The gain achieved is therefore theoretically much the same, but pollicisation leaves scars in the palm and some impairment of function in the middle and little fingers. If the index finger is pollicised, the benefit of the operation is still less since this finger is worth 20 per cent.

In total amputations, a pollicised index finger will make a thumb worth 20 to 25 per cent, the overall gain therefore being 0 to 5 per cent. Reconstruction by tube pedicle gives a thumb worth only 10 per cent. The benefit is thus about the same with both procedures.

SUBTOTAL LOSS OF THE THUMB

The good results obtained in cases of subtotal loss of the thumb when the tube pedicle and bone graft method is used, indicate to us that the main functional needs are met. We would only consider pollicisation justified where the patient needs to undertake particularly precise and fine work or for cosmetic reasons. In this case, we prefer to use the ring finger because the sacrifice is less.

TOTAL LOSS OF THE THUMB

In total amputation, pollicisation of the index finger whether intact or partially amputated, is the best method of thumb reconstruction. If the index finger also is amputated at metacarpophalangeal joint level, or more proximally, deepening of the first web may be combined with pollicisation of the index stump. If this is not possible, pollicisation of one of the three intact remaining digits is too much of a sacrifice for the quality of grasp. Reconstruction by tube pedicle and bone graft should then be performed.

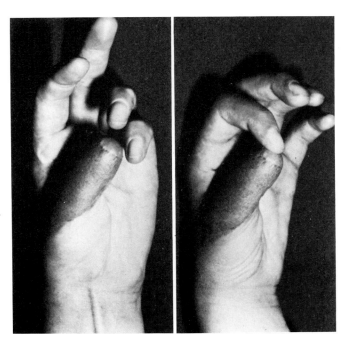

Figure 16.6
The reconstructed thumb has a satisfactory appearance and a good function.

CONCLUSION

A wide knowledge of the possibilities and limitations of this method of thumb reconstruction should enable one to select suitable cases for operation. We look upon pollicisation and tube pedicle/bone graft reconstruction as two particular methods of thumb reconstruction which may be applied to different specific situations, not necessarily as alternatives to be considered in every case.

BIBLIOGRAPHY

LITTLER, J. W. (1956). Neurovascular pedicle transfer of tissue in reconstructive surgery of the hand. *Journal of Bone and Joint Surgery*, **38-A,** 917.

McGREGOR, I. A. & SIMONETTA, C. (1964). Reconstruction of thumb by composite bone–skin flap. *British Journal of Plastic Surgery*, **17,** 37.

McGREGOR, I. A. & JACKSON, I. T. (1971). The groin flap. *British Journal of Plastic Surgery*, **24,** 3.

MOBERG, E. (1955). *Journal of Bone and Joint Surgery*, **37A,** 307.

NICOLADONI, C. (1900). Daumenplastik und organischer Ersatz der Fingerspitze (Anticheiroplastik und Daktyloplastik). *Archiv für Klinische Chirurgie*, **61,** 606.

SIMONETTA, C. (1973). Simplifications et améliorations de la technique de reconstruction du pouce. *Congrès Européen de Chirurgie plastique*, Madrid, 1973.

SIMONETTA, C. (1975). Chirurgie réparatrice des pertes de substance et des amputations du pouce. *Thèse présentée à la Faculté de Médecine de Lausanne.*

TUBIANA, R. & DUPARC, J. (1960). Un procédé nouveau de reconstruction d'un pouce sensible (Rapport de R. Merle d'Aubigné). *Mémoires de l'Académie de Chirurgie*, **86,** 264–268.

17. RECONSTRUCTION OF THE MUTILATED HAND USING MICROSURGERY

A. Gilbert and R. Tubiana

Transplantation of bone, sensitive skin and intact digits using microsurgical techniques has opened new vistas of reconstruction for the hand surgeon. We do not intend to discuss the techniques of microsurgical nerve repair here. Microsurgical techniques have been available for 15 years but the clinical applications have only recently become feasible. Cobbett in 1969 published the first description of a free graft of the big toe to reconstruct the thumb. However, one had to wait until 1974 to find the first description of a free groin flap applied to the hand (O'Brien *et al.* and Harii *et al.*) and it was only in 1976 that transfer of the second toe (Ohmorii) and the first neurovascular flap from the pulp of the toes (Gilbert *et al.*) were described.

Thus it is fair to say that all these series have a very short follow-up. It is only possible to get some idea of the very early results. We will have to wait some years to judge the long-term results of these procedures.

1. RECONSTRUCTION OF THE SKIN

There are two indications for major skin reconstruction. The first is to restore skin following a burn or avulsion. This is most commonly seen on the dorsum of the hand. The second is for replacement of scars and contractures affecting web spaces. We are not suggesting this technique as a substitution for all free grafts to the hand but rather as an alternative to pedicle flaps. The advantages of doing this are as follows.

The entire procedure is completed at one operation. This removes the need to immobilise the hand in a difficult position. It allows the hand to be elevated immediately and enables the patient to start early movements. There is less risk of infection as the hand may be kept dry and this means there is less risk in undertaking other procedures such as osteotomy, tendon or bone grafts. Hospitalisation is much shorter and there is an earlier return to activity. However, one cannot ignore the deficiencies of this method. Firstly, the operation is prolonged (4–6 hours). Secondly, the technique may not be possible due to adverse local conditions, e.g. if the prospective recipient site has an inadequate blood supply. Finally there is the possibility of complications. These are uncommon but represent a risk of between 10 and 15 per cent (Harii, 1975; Gilbert and Dessapt, 1976).

There should be a very good reason for using this technique in a situation where a pedicle flap is possible. A free flap should only be used where direct pedicle flaps are either impossible or where there is urgent need for comfort, asepsis and early re-education. Once the indications have been established there are several types of free flap available.

1. *The groin flap* (McGregor, 1972). This is the flap most frequently used in a free flap transfer and has a number of advantages: (1) large size; (2) a vascular pedicle which is relatively constant and of a reasonable size (1–1·2 mm), and (3) an adequate cosmetic result as the scar is within the bikini area. The disadvantages of this site: (1) the thickness of the flap particularly in a fat patient, and (2) absence of sensation. Its use therefore is reserved solely for large skin defects of the hand and it is not used in pressure areas.

2. *The free flap from the dorsum of the foot* (McGraw, 1975). This flap is supplied by the cutaneous branches of the dorsalis pedis artery. It requires a delicate technique to raise the flap but it does have certain advantages. It is thin; and its pedicle is long and of adequate size. Finally and above all it can be provided with sensation by incorporating the terminal branches of the musculo-cutaneous nerve. The sensibility that this produces is only of a protective nature but may be utilised for example, in the web spaces of the hand. There are, however, two disadvantages. It is of small size (in the region of 10×8 cm) and the loss of substance on the foot must be grafted, occasionally at a second operation.

3. *The free flap from the web spaces of the foot* (Gilbert, 1975). This flap is made up of skin which most closely resembles that of the hand and it possesses both a vascular and nerve pedicle that are well defined (Gilbert, 1976). It comprises the 1st web space and the pulps from the adjacent halves of the toes. It has certain advantages. Firstly, its texture and sensation are very similar to that of the fingers. Secondly, its shape adapts it perfectly for use in the thumb/index web space. There is a small defect at the donor site and this may be grafted. There are some disadvantages. It involves a difficult dissection. The flap may easily be extended on the dorsum of the foot but not on the plantar surface. This flap is virtually only used in the hand where it is required to provide sensation following severe injuries. It may also be used either simply as a free flap for the 1st web space following correction of an adducted thumb, or to provide a single pulp.

These three flaps are the ones most commonly used. There are others, for example a delto-pectoral or axillary flap but they are rarely used.

THE OPERATION

1. The preparation of the recipient site is made by a separate team. The scar is excised, any orthopaedic procedures undertaken and the pedicles prepared. Usually the

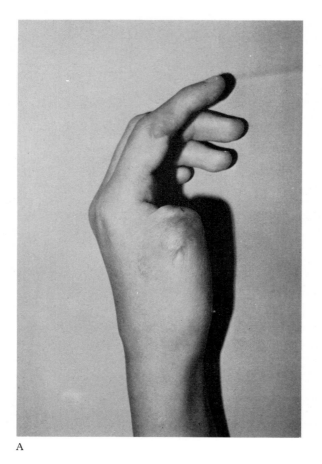

A

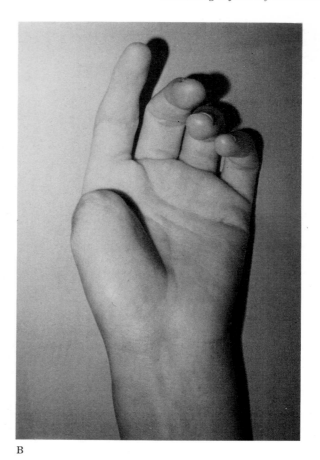

B

Figure 17.1
Loss of thumb at metacarpophalangeal joint level.

anastomoses are performed on the dorsum of the hand. The artery most commonly used is the dorsal branch of the radial artery. It may, in fact, be used even if it was injured in the original trauma. It is first necessary to apply Allen's test or arteriography with compression (Doyon, 1976) to make sure that there will be an adequate blood supply to the rest of the hand. It is usually easy to find a vein on the dorsum of the hand for reconstructions of the web space. The nerve used is a dorsal branch of the radial nerve and for a pulp the corresponding digital bundle is used too. During this time the second team prepare the free flap. First of all the vascular pedicle is isolated to make sure of its existence and size. The flap is then elevated. As a third stage of the procedure the first team now closes or grafts the donor site whilst the second team places the flap and anastomoses the vessels. The microscope is used (magnification of between 10 and 30 times) to anastomose the vessels with 10 zero sutures. The arterial anastomosis is done first to reduce the ischaemia time, the flap remaining devascularised, on average 30 to 50 minutes. Light dressings are applied to allow observation of the distal part every half hour. The patient is in hospital for 15 to 20 days.

2. DIGITAL RECONSTRUCTION

Reconstruction of a complete thumb by transfer of a toe with vascular anastomosis is only a modern application of a very ancient technique. Nicoladoni described the principle in 1895 and actually performed it in 1898. Since then some dozens of cases have been done with diverse results. Despite the fact that it gives satisfactory results (Clarkson 1962, Freeman 1965) the method of transfer by pedicle flap has fallen into disuse basically because of the uncomfortable position which has to be assumed by the patient. This position is very difficult to maintain and, in fact, often has to be abandoned. This accounts for a number of the complications of this technique. It is for this reason that the technique has been discontinued, not because of poor cosmetic or functional results. Clarkson has shown that in 13 of his patients 15 years after the operation there was no functional disability in the foot. For this reason the technique was re-instituted in a simplified form using a direct vascularised transfer from the toe to the hand. Cobbett performed this in 1969 and since then about 30 cases have been reported in the world literature. Complications are rare when the vascular anatomy of the toes is fully appreciated. Their arterial supply arises basically from the dorsalis pedis artery via the dorsal interosseous branch in the first space.

PREOPERATIVE PREPARATION

It is necessary to delineate the vascular supply accurately as it is subject to a number of variations. Palpation or ultrasound will enable one to establish the presence of an artery in the first space but only arteriography will confirm its position with absolute certainty. This information makes the operation both easier and shorter.

The second important part of the preparation is choice of toe. The first or second may be transplanted with equal ease. They are both dependent upon the same vascular supply. The decision therefore is usually made in conjunction with the patient, taking into consideration his occupation and his feelings about the final appearance.

The big toe presents certain advantages over the second: (1) it allows reconstruction of a thumb which is both more solid and more aesthetic, and (2) its flexor tendon may be dissected out for a sufficient length to enable suture at the level of the wrist. It does, however, have some disadvantages.

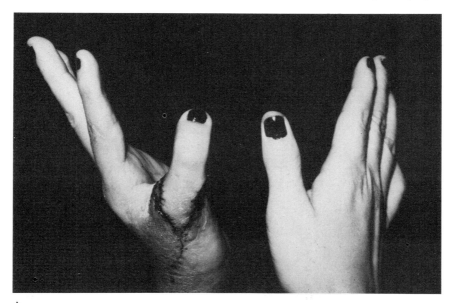

A

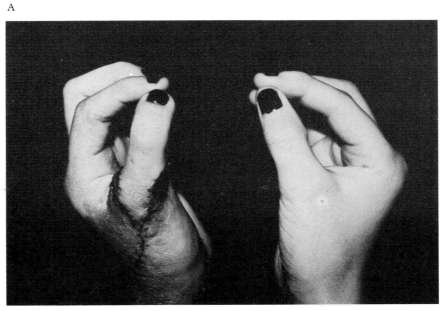

B

Figure 17.2
Result of free transfer of the 2nd toe.

Its absence from the foot is more noticeable and the functional disability is greater than after the removal of the second toe. It cannot be taken with part of the 1st metatarsal therefore. If there is an indication for it, the 2nd metatarsal may be taken with the 2nd toe. In nearly all the cases which have been published to date it is the big toe which has been chosen for reconstruction of the thumb. In our series 12 of 15 transplanted toes were second toes.

If one applies purely cosmetic considerations then reconstruction of the distal part of a digit is performed by using the terminal phalanx of the 2nd toe along with its nail or even just the pulp itself (Buncke 1975).

THE OPERATION

This follows the same principles as for the free-flap transfer using two teams. The anastomoses are usually done on the dorsum of the hand at the level of the anatomical snuff box. It is an advantage to place the tendon sutures as far proximal as possible.

Fixation is either by an arthrodesis done by resecting the base of the proximal phalanx or if the head of the 1st metacarpal is preserved one can form a new metacarpophalangeal joint. The base of the proximal phalanx of the thumb is excised but the capsule including the articular fibrocartilage is preserved. The toe is taken with the dorsal and lateral capsule of the metatarsophalangeal joint. The suture of this capsule to the remaining structures in the thumb provides adequate stability and osteosynthesis is unnecessary. It is thus possible to preserve some mobility at this level. Finally the digital nerves are sutured to those of the thumb. Everything must be done in one procedure to avoid having to re-operate. Surgery in the region of a vascular anastomosis is delicate and dangerous.

The final stage is skin closure which often poses problems and needs meticulous preoperative planning. Complete closure is usually possible when an arthrodesis has been performed because the phalanx of the toe has been shortened. In other circumstances there is usually a persistent skin defect. This defect is usually minimal and is often located on the dorso-ulnar aspect of the transplanted digit. Provided the vessels are satisfactorily covered a skin graft may well be adequate. If, however, important structures such as tendons or vessels are exposed, it is necessary to use a local flap, e.g., from the index finger. In some cases (amputation at the base of the metacarpal or severe scarring) the loss of skin is considerable. Several authors (Tsai 1975, Millesi 1976) have used abdominal flaps at the same operation. In such cases we prefer to use a pedicle flap at a first operation followed by the transfer of the toe 3 weeks later.

POSTOPERATIVE CARE

A padded dressing is used leaving the pulp of the toe exposed. Postoperative treatment is simple comprising (1) antibiotics, (2) aspirin, (3) dypyramidole (Persantin). Close observation is continued for about 20 days. Very gentle mobilisation is begun at an early stage.

THE RESULTS

At the present time there are few published results. Most of these have been satisfactory. Cosmetically the operation gives good results with a large thumb possessing a nail. The functional results depend to a large extent on the preoperative condition particularly the level of amputation. When the thumb loss is at metacarpophalangeal joint level with preservation of the thenar muscles the results are excellent (as with all other reconstructive procedures). (Figs. 17.1 to 17.3).

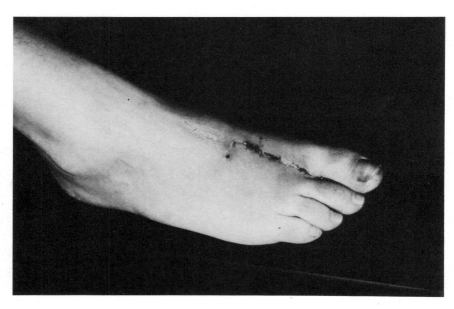

Figure 17.3
Satisfactory appearance of foot following removal of 2nd toe.

Sensory return is similar to that following a digital nerve repair—that is to say satisfactory but never perfect.

INDICATIONS

These follow on from the previous paragraph. The best indication for this reconstruction is when the thumb has been amputated at the level of the metacarpophalangeal joint. One can almost always predict satisfactory results in these cases. The operation is also possible in cases of total amputation of the thumb and metacarpal. In our opinion the only indication for this procedure in such cases is where the alternative methods are contra-indicated.

Finally it must be added that the wishes and motivation of the patient are fundamental. He may refuse a mutilation of the foot and prefer to lose one of the four remaining fingers.

This method is obviously only one technique available to the hand surgeon. It will fall into disrepute if it is used indiscriminately and should only be considered together with the other techniques available.

BIBLIOGRAPHY

BUNCKE, H. J. (1975). Digital transplantation. *Clinics in Plastic Surgery*, p. 295.

CLARCKSON, P. (1962). On making thumbs. *Plastic and Reconstructive Surgery*, **29**, 325.

COBBETT, J. R. (1969). Free digital transfer. *Journal of Bone and Joint Surgery*, **51B**, 577.

FREEMAN, B. (1965). Reconstruction of the thumb by toe transfer. *Plastic and Reconstructive Surgery*, **17**, 393.

GILBERT, A., MORRISON, W. A., TUBIANA, R., LISFRANC, R. & FIRMIN, F. (1975). Transfert sur la main d'un lambeau libre sensible. *Chirurgie*, **101**, 621.

GILBERT, A. (1976). Composite tissue transfers from the foot. In *Symposium on Microsurgery*, p. 230. MOSBY.

GILBERT, A. & DESSAPT, B. (1976). Lambeaux libres avec micro-anastomoses vasculaires. *Chirurgie*, **102**, 980.

HARII, K., OHMORI, K. & OHMORI, S. (1974). Successful clinical transfer of ten free flaps by microvascular anastomosis. *Plastic and Reconstructive Surgery*, **53**, 259.

HARII, K., OHMORI, K., TORII, S., MURAKAMI, F., KASAI, Y., SEKIGUHI, J. & OHMORI, S. (1975). Free groin flaps. *British Journal of Plastic Surgery*, **28**, 225.

MACCRAW, J. & FURLOW, L. (1975). The dorsalis pedis arterialized flap. *Plastic and Reconstructive Surgery*, **55**, 177.

MACGREGOR, I. A. & JACKSON, I. T. (1972). The groin flap. *British Journal of Plastic Surgery*, **25**, 3.

MILLESI, H. (1976). Personal communication.

O'BRIEN, B. McC., MORRISON, W. A., ISHIDA, H., MACLEOD, A. M. & GILBERT, A. (1974). Free flap transfers with microvascular anastomoses. *British Journal of Plastic Surgery*, **27**, 220.

OHMORI, K. & HARII, K. (1975). Transplantation of a toe to an amputated finger. *Hand*, **7**, 134.

TSAI, T. (1975). Experimental and clinical applications of microvascular surgery. *Annals of Surgery*, **181**, 169.

H

18. DIGITAL RECONSTRUCTION BY MICROSURGICAL TRANSFER OF THE SECOND TOE

C. le Quang, P. Banzet and C. Dufourmentel

Cobbett (1969), Buncke (1966) and O'Brien (1975) have been responsible for introducing new techniques in hand reconstruction using microsurgical techniques to transfer the big toe at one operation. Then Ohmori and Harii published for the first time in 1975 the case of microsurgical transfer of the 2nd toe to elongate a damaged index finger. Cobbett uses one of the plantar collateral vessels for the pedicle of the big toe while Buncke and O'Brien use the terminal branch of the dorsalis pedis artery which usually branches both to the 1st and 2nd toes. Ohmori and Harii use the same vessels for taking the 2nd toe.

We shall describe the technique of transferring the 2nd toe to the hand, this being taken with a dorsalis pedis pedicle and anastomosed to the radial artery on the dorsum of the hand whether the thumb or index finger is being reconstructed.

OPERATIVE TECHNIQUE

1. Preoperative arteriography is essential. It should be undertaken within two weeks of operation. It provides information on the vascularisation of both the hand and the foot. In the hand by compression of the radial artery one can

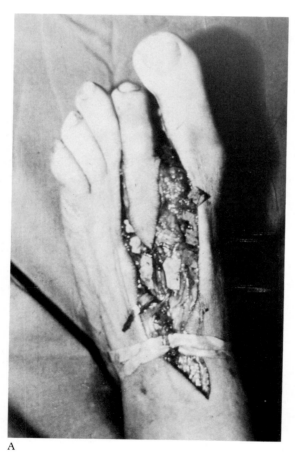

A

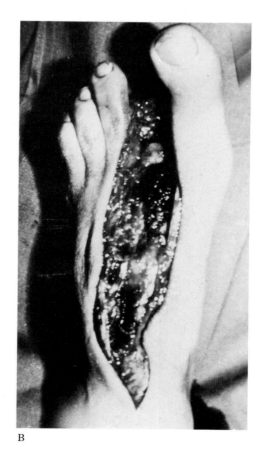

B

Figure 18.1

A, Mobilising the 2nd toe. Incision on the dorsum of the foot exposing the superficial veins and the dorsalis pedis pedicle. Note the skin flap raised in continuity with the toe.

B, After mobilising the 2nd toe one can see the head of the 2nd metatarsal which has been partially removed to aid closure of the gap.

assess the adequacy of the circulation from the ulnar artery before using the former for the anastomosis.

In the foot one can confirm the presence of a dorsalis pedis artery and its first interosseous branch supplying both the big and second toes. At the same time one can confirm that there will be adequate circulation to the remaining toes via the plantar anastomoses.

2. The operation is started by taking the 2nd toe under tourniquet control. The dorsalis pedis artery is dissected out to the level of the extensor retinaculum (Fig. 18.1) and is then ligatured at its termination at the base of the first interspace as it gives rise to the first dorsal interosseous. This vessel is then mobilised to the base of the 2nd toe, taking with it more or less muscle depending on whether it lies superficial or deep in the intermetatarsal space. By taking the dorsalis pedis and its branch in the 1st interspace one can produce a pedicle in the region of 15 cm. Two veins are identified. The first is the deep vein from the dorsum of the foot that forms part of the dorsal venous arch. It is possible to take a long dorsal skin flap based on the same vascular pedicle. The other structures identified and raised are the extensor tendons and the branch of the musculocutaneous nerve.

On the plantar surface a long zig-zag incision is made proximally towards the arch which allows isolation of the 1st and 2nd plantar digital arteries. At the level of the bifurcation the collateral vessels to the 2nd toe are tied, then the digital nerves are dissected out and the branches to the 2nd toe are cut. Each nerve is cut as far back as possible. At the same time the flexor tendons are dissected out and cut as far posteriorly in the arch as possible.

A small triangle of plantar skin is taken in continuity with the 2nd toe which is finally detached either through the metatarsophalangeal joint or by osteotomy of the neck of the metatarsal if the head is to be taken to provide an articular reconstruction (Fig. 18.2). Before cutting the dorsalis pedis artery, the tourniquet is removed to confirm that the blood supply of the 2nd toe on this vessel is adequate.

The preparation of the hand is also done under tourniquet. On the dorsal surface the structures exposed are the radial artery accompanied by its veins at the level of the anatomical snuff box, a subcutaneous vein either to the thumb or another finger, a dorsal branch of the radial nerve and the extensor tendon. On the palmar aspect both digital nerves are isolated and the flexor tendons exposed at the level of the wrist.

The detached 2nd toe is bathed in heparinised saline and transferred to the hand. After osteosynthesis by two crossed wires the end-to-end microvascular anastomoses are made using 9 or 10 zero nylon. The dorsalis pedis is anastomosed to the radial artery on the dorsum of the hand and both the veins are anastomosed if possible. The dorsalis pedis vein is anastomosed to the vein accompanying the radial artery and the superficial vein to one on the other side. The tourniquet is released between the arterial and venous anastomoses to confirm adequate filling of the artery and a return flow in the veins.

The tendons are sutured preferably at the level of the wrist and certainly as far as possible from the vascular and nerve anastomoses. It is essential to repair an extensor and a flexor tendon and this is done by side-to-side anastomosis with an overlap of 2 cm using simple nylon sutures. This gives a sound union and allows early mobilisation.

The nerve anastomosis is also done under the microscope with 10 or 11 zero nylon. On the dorsum of the hand the terminal branch of the musculocutaneous is anastomosed to the digital branch of the radial nerve. On the palmar surface the two digital nerves are anastomosed. If the nerves of the toe are very small then it is necessary simply to put both collateral nerve endings into one of the digital nerves. It is vital to avoid any tension even having an excess of length if necessary.

Finally after very careful haemostasis the skin is sutured leaving a rubber drain, haematoma being a common cause of early thrombosis. The strip of skin taken from the dorsum of the foot means that the dorsal incision on the hand can be closed without tension. It is preferable however to put split-skin grafts around the edge of this skin strip rather than to risk tension on the anastomosis by attempting straight wound suture.

The foot is closed simply by approximating the big and 3rd toes after having resected the head of the 2nd metatarsal.

3. Postoperatively the hand is elevated at the level of the patient's heart. An intravenous infusion of Reomacrodex

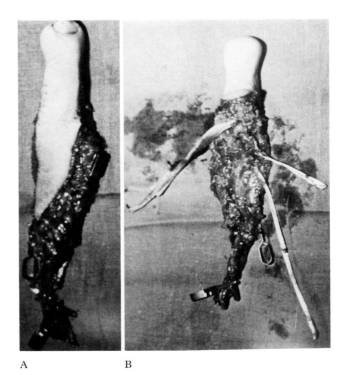

A   B

Figure 18.2
The isolated 2nd toe.
A, A view from the dorsal aspect with the skin flap.
B, The plantar view with the tendons and long vascular pedicle in a clamp (1 artery and 2 veins).

which is started two days before the operation continues for five to seven days. This is in addition to vasodilators (Persantin and aspirin) which are used over a period of two or three weeks. Smoking is forbidden for several months. We do not usually give heparin. Active physiotherapy starts during the second week and becomes more intensive after removal of the wires between the thirtieth and forty-fifth days. Sensation in the pulp reappears around the third or fourth month at about the same time as there is functional return.

CLINICAL RESULTS

We have performed to date, six transfers of the 2nd toe to the hand. On four occasions this was to reconstruct the thumb and twice to reconstruct the index finger.

1. From a technical point of view we have been able to utilise, in five cases, the dorsalis pedis artery and the radial artery. In one case, in a reconstruction of the thumb, the dorsalis pedis was short with absence of the first interosseous bifurcation and in that case we used one of the plantar arteries and part of the arch which gave origin to it. The

dissection in the plantar fat was very difficult and the length of the pedicle was less than 5 cm which meant that we had to perform the anastomosis in the palm with a branch of the superficial palmar arch. This made the operation much more difficult and we were using vessels in the region of 1 to 1·5 mm compared with the dorsalis pedis which is, on average, in the region of 2 to 3 mm.

2. In terms of survival of the transplant, we have had no complication as a result of arterial thrombosis. In one case a venous thrombosis necessitated re-operation on the third day. This was in a case where only one venous anastomosis had been performed and although the operation produced adequate venous drainage, it served to emphasise the necessity of having two venous anastomoses.

3. We can only comment on the functional result of our two earliest cases which we have followed-up for more than a year.

Mr. L., aged 21, a locksmith, had a transfer of the 2nd toe for amputation of the thumb of the left hand at the level of the metacarpophalangeal joint (Fig. 18.3). At 14 months he had practically normal function of the new thumb with two-point discrimination in the pulp of 10 mm. Pulp-to-pulp opposition

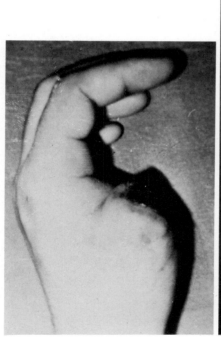
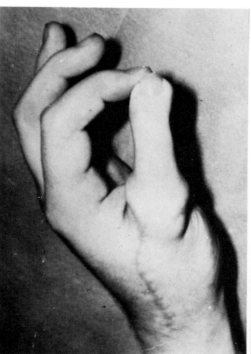
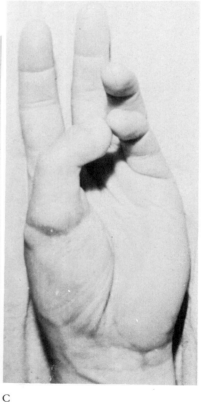

A   B   C

Figure 18.3
Transfer of the 2nd toe for a thumb.
A, Amputation of the left thumb over the metacarpophalangeal joint.
B and C, Result at one year showing opposition of the new thumb with the index and the little finger.

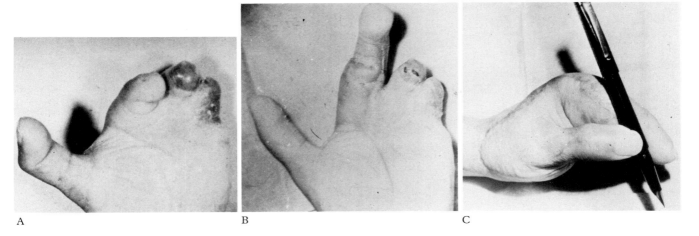

A   B   C

Figure 18.4
Transfer of the 2nd toe for the index.
A, Proximal amputation of the four fingers of the left hand.
B and C, Result at one year showing the new index in extension (B) and in pinch with the thumb (C).

was possible to all the fingers. There were no problems with the foot and he had returned to his job at six months.

Mr. P., aged 39, a mechanic, had a transfer of the 2nd left toe to reconstruct the left index finger following amputation of all the fingers at the level of the mid-part of the proximal phalanges (Fig. 18.4). At 12 months he had two-point discrimination in the pulp of 12 mm and a good pinch between the thumb and index finger. There were no problems with the foot and he returned to work at six months after industrial retraining as a warehouse man.

4. Finally, from the cosmetic point of view, replacement of the thumb with the 2nd toe gives a surprisingly good result compared with the use of the great toe, which sometimes gives the appearance of macrodactyly. Transfer of the 2nd toe has little effect on the foot either from a functional or cosmetic point of view, contrasting with the result of transferring the big toe (Fig. 18.5).

CONCLUSIONS

We believe that the technique of microsurgical transfer of the 2nd toe is now well established but accept that it is still subject to all the complications of microvascular surgery. However, use of the dorsalis pedis and radial artery which have a reasonable size, seems to produce good viability. Using the technique in a sensible fashion one can obtain a digit of reasonable appearance and satisfactory sensation, even if the mobility is not perfect. The operation can produce a sensitive pinch grip either in reconstructing a thumb amputated at the level of the metacarpophalangeal joint (particularly when the thenar muscles are preserved) or in reconstructing an index finger where only the thumb remains following amputation at the level of the proximal phalanges or metacarpophalangeal joints.

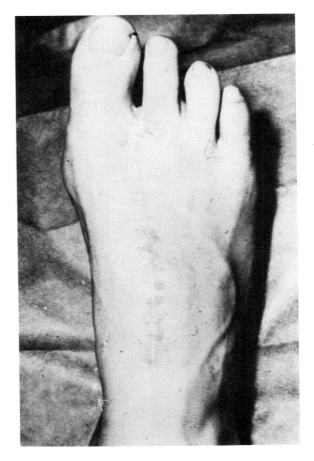

Figure 18.5
Dorsal view of the foot one year after removal of the 2nd toe.

This technique must always be measured against the classical methods of reconstructing the thumb in any particular situation.

BIBLIOGRAPHY

BUNCKE, H. J., BUNCKE, C. M., & SCHULZ, W. P. (1966). Immediate Nicoladoni procedure in the Rhesus monkey, or hallux-to-hand transplantation utilising microminiature vascular anastomosis. *British Journal of Plastic Surgery*, **19,** 332.

BUNCKE, H. J., McLEAN, D. H., GEROGE, P. T., CREECH, B. J. & CHATER, N. L. (1973). Thumb replacement: Great toe transplantation by microvascular anastomosis. *British Journal of Plastic Surgery*, **26,** 194.

BUNCKE, H. J. (1975). Free toe-to-hand transplantations by micro-vascular anastomosis. *Transactions of the Sixth International Congress of Plastic and Reconstructive Surgery*, Paris, p. 69.

COBBETT, J. R. (1969). Free digital transfer: Report of a case of transfer of a great toe to replace an amputated thumb. *Journal of Bone and Joint Surgery*, **51-B,** 677.

GILBERT, A. (1976). Composite tissue transfers from the foot: anatomic basis and surgical technique. *Proceedings of the International Symposium on Micro-Surgery*, ed. Daniller, A. and Strauch, B., Saint Louis, 230.

LE QUANG, C., BANZET, P. & SERVANT, J. M. (1976). Reconstruction du pouce et de l'index par transposition du 2me orteil avec micro-anastomoses vasculo nerveuses *Communication au XXI° Congrès de la Société Française de Chirurgie Plastique et Reconstructive*, Biarritz, 29 juin 1976.

O'BRIEN, B. McC., MacLEOD, A. M., SYKES, P. J. & DONAHOE, S. (1975). Hallux-to-hand transfer. *The Hand*, **7,** 128.

OHMORI, K. & HARII, K. (1975). Transplantation of a toe to an amputated finger. *The Hand*, **7,** 134.

19. SECONDARY TENOLYSIS AFTER POLLICISATION

J. Michon

Pollicisation of a finger is, in our opinion, only justified when it results in a thumb possessing normal power and independent action, and as full a range of motion as possible in addition to normal sensibility. The necessary conditions for achieving a satisfactory result depend to a large extent on the preoperative condition of the hand and the technique used in the transfer. The basic techniques, and particularly the choice of tendons used for producing extension, have been described by more authoritative exponents than ourselves. Assuming that the objective with regard to sensibility has been achieved, a critical review of our results, made in close collaboration with a rehabilitation centre, has, from our very first case, demonstrated certain frequent deficiencies in pollicisation regarding motor function: deficient metacarpophalangeal extension and limitation of flexion both in amplitude and power. Functional tests at the centre have shown that these defects could prevent a patient from being able to return to certain exacting types of manual work.

We have been particularly struck by a variant of the syndrome whereby independent action of the digits does not occur due to linkage of the profundus tendons. When the thumb has been reconstructed by transferring the ring finger, flexion of the thumb is accompanied by simultaneous flexion of the middle finger and *vice versa*. If the middle finger has been used for the reconstruction then the ring finger is affected in the same way. This has produced good spherical prehension in grasping but independent functioning is not so good.

These considerations have led us to operate again on certain patients and the findings at operation have confirmed the following points:

1. *Extension lag* is largely avoidable by a correct re-creation of the extensor apparatus of the transferred finger. If it is necessary to reinforce the central slip (e.g. by extensor pollicis longus), it is also necessary to reinforce the two lateral slips. Without this precaution, extension of the distal two segments can never be complete. For this procedure we have available, basically, the thenar muscles, but they are not always present or in a satisfactory functioning state. One can replace them with adjacent long tendons e.g. extensor pollicis brevis, extensor of a transferred finger which has been discarded or extensor indicis. Even if the tendon junctions have been correctly established it is still possible for adhesions to prevent active extension or to prevent full flexion.

2. *Lack of flexion* may be explained, to a large extent, by the lack of independent action in the flexor tendons of the transferred finger. We know that there is considerable linkage between the flexor tendons at the wrist and in the carpal tunnel giving joint action of the fingers. Pollicisation does not alter this arrangement and it is impossible to remedy it at the primary operation without hazarding the blood supply of the transferred finger.

Added to this there is also the lack of tension in the flexor tendon of the transferred finger when either index or middle finger is used and the aim is to produce a thumb of normal length without amputating the distal phalanx.

On the other hand, flexor tendon adhesions only occasionally account for the lack of flexion if one has taken care to preserve intact the fibrous flexor sheath in the course of the dissection.

We have found by experience that it is possible to rectify the various deficiencies of pollicisation by a secondary intervention. This can be undertaken 3 to 4 months after the reconstruction when scarring, tendon junctions and the bony fusion are stable and when there is no longer any further increase in active movements.

If there is lack of active extension at the level of the metacarpophalangeal joint of the thumb, we undertake a revision of the three anastomoses by tenolysis at a time when this is always a simple and straightforward procedure.

To improve flexion we open the wrist and carpal tunnel and free the flexors of the new thumb from their connections as far proximally as the muscle bellies to give them maximal independence of action realising, of course, that at the muscle level their contractions can never be completely dissociated. For this reason, in addition to this freeing procedure, we also attach the flexor pollicis longus, provided it is usable, to the flexor profundus of the pollicised digit in the lower part of the forearm. The tension in this reinforcing tendon should be greater than the existing tension in the flexor profundus to overcome its lack of tension and to improve the cortical control of movement and of the finger in its new position. This tendon transfer must not interfere with immediate mobilisation: an interlacing type of tendon junction over a distance of several centimetres will allow this.

The aim of this secondary procedure is, therefore, freeing of the motors of the new thumb enabling it to develop considerable independent action.

It cannot, of course, be considered as an essential measure and undertaken in all patients who have had a pollicisation.

The indications for this are relative and reserved for young patients whose work necessitates manual dexterity. It is also necessary that candidates for this operation should be keen and have shown that they have the necessary ability to rehabilitate themselves. Finally, it is imperative that the pollicised finger should have a perfect blood supply, absence of trophic changes and normal sensibility, to obviate any risk by a further operative procedure.

Postoperative management : the main feature is the institution at an early stage of active movements, in practice from the fourth day, after removal of the Redon drain. The attachment of the flexor pollicis longus tendon does not prevent this, since, being interlaced over a distance of several centimetres, it provides a strong anastomosis and may be mobilised at once.

The results have, in all cases, been very encouraging, as evidenced by a rapid gain in amplitude of movement but above all by a much more 'automatic' action of the thumb. Photographs fail to demonstrate the true gain in function. The patients' appreciation is, for us, the major factor which

has encouraged us to pursue this line of treatment in spite of one's dislike, in principle, of repeated procedures.

Contra-indications : secondary tenolysis is contra-indicated if one has reason to think that the tendons of the transferred digit have a poor blood supply. In one of our patients where a ring finger had been pollicised after a serious hand injury with multiple lesions of tendons, nerves and vessels, tenolysis was undertaken as far as the digit, with removal of the flexor superficialis in addition. In the course of re-education the tendon ruptured necessitating a flexor tendon graft. The end result was acceptable but reminded us of the need for caution in these complicated cases.

20. COMMENTS ON A MUTILATED THUMB

D. Morel-Fatio

On the 9th August 1966, the manager of a farming estate was involved in an accident; his right thumb was crushed by the helicoid screw of a harvester. The local surgeon, realising the seriousness of the injury and the difficulty of deciding immediately about the viability of the damaged tissues, proceeded to suture the skin flaps and immobilise the multiple fractures of the thumb in a functional position using a plaster incorporating hand and forearm. A month later the dressing was taken down for the first time. The whole of the volar aspect was necrotic.

We examined the patient on the 25th September, 6 weeks after the accident. The sum total of damage was as follows (Figs. 20.1 and 20.2).

Skin: necrosis over the volar aspect of the proximal and distal phalanges of the thumb.

Tendons: on lifting the slough, the flexor pollicis longus was also found to be necrotic.

Neurovascular bundles: both bundles had been avulsed, with complete sensory loss over the thumb pulp and on either side of the necrotic area. The extensor aspect was normal but threatened at the base of the thumb by the protrusion of a metacarpal bone splinter.

Skeletal structure: the base of the 1st metacarpal was intact together with its muscle attachments providing good active movements in all directions. The greater part of the 1st metacarpal had been detached as a long fragment, the point of which threatened to penetrate the skin of the dorsum.

The proximal phalanx had been fractured through its middle, the proximal segment was exposed, but the distal part, the interphalangeal joint and the distal phalanx seemed intact.

There was no active movement at the interphalangeal joint.

When the slough was removed, granulation tissue was seen which, on bacteriological examination, revealed growth of staphylococcus aureus, sensitive to current antibiotics.

What line of treatment should be adopted in these circumstances?

ACCEPT THE THUMB AS A WRITE-OFF AND AMPUTATE IT THROUGH THE 1ST METACARPAL, WITH A VIEW TO UNDERTAKING POLLICISATION LATER

If one wished to make a thumb with mobile joints, one could consider this possibility, but in this particular case we decided against it.

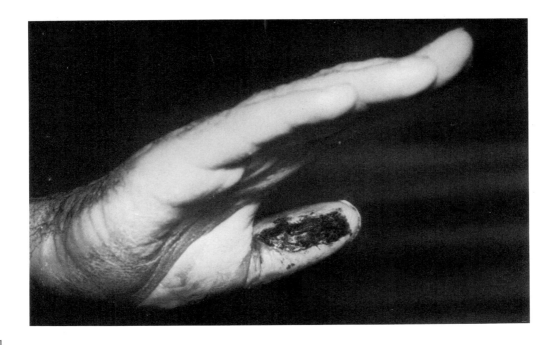

Figure 20.1

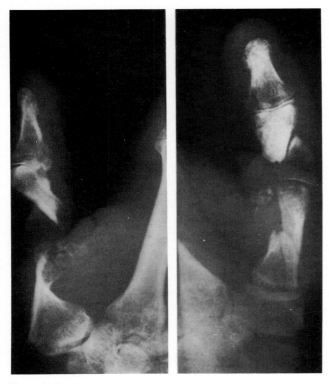

Figure 20.2

PRESERVE THE MUTILATED THUMB AND ATTEMPT TO REPAIR IT

Two essential facts must be noted:

This thumb was considerably shortened, 6 weeks having elapsed since the accident.

There was no function of the interphalangeal joint owing to sloughing of the flexor tendon and shortening of the digit which caused an extensor tendon lag.

1. *Should one try to preserve an intact interphalangeal joint?*
This ideal aim would assume:

If one wished to restore extension, it would be essential to restore the digit to its normal length to provide the long extensor tendon with its original tone. If, however, this was not possible due to contracture of the soft tissues there was no question of restoring length. Extensor function must definitely be considered lost unless one shortens the long extensor later and the results of this are most uncertain.

If one wishes to restore flexion, it would be necessary to do a secondary tendon graft after having bone-grafted the defect between base of metacarpal and base of proximal phalanx. It would therefore be necessary to resurface the volar aspect with a flap having subcutaneous tissue to provide for gliding action of the tendon. This could only be achieved by a distant flap and would therefore lack sensation.

All this would involve a minimum of four operations and achieve in the end a doubtful result, a thumb with pulp lacking sensation and an interphalangeal joint which would undoubtedly be stiff or unstable.

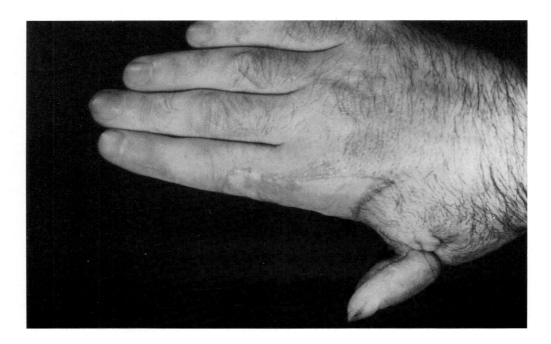

Figure 20.3

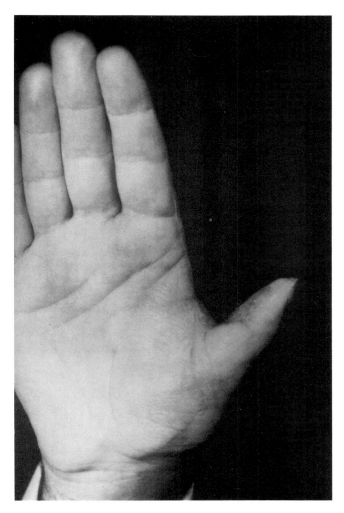

Figure 20.4

strict aseptic conditions. This delay will certainly lead to more shortening of the thumb but we have seen that, far from being a disadvantage, this is our aim.

First operation: 29th September 1966, 7 weeks after the accident. The necrotic area which included sloughing flexor tendon was removed, together with all dead tissue. Bone sequestrum which included the greater part of the metacarpal extending distally to the proximal phalanx was also removed. The skin defect was replaced by a local flap raised on the radial and dorsal aspects of the index finger based proximally. This long and relatively narrow flap was let into the base of the thumb and covered the volar aspect without tension or kinking. A split-skin graft was used to cover the donor site on the index finger. Postoperative course was apyrexial, viability of the flap was entirely satisfactory and all dressings were dispensed with after 3 weeks. The condition of the hand after the first operation is shown (Figs. 20.3 and 20.4). The furrow on the back of the thumb can be seen.

Second operation was undertaken on 7th February 1967, 4 months after the first. A bone graft was taken from the anterior end of the right iliac crest (2/3 cortical bone and 1/3 cancellous). The thumb was approached through its dorsal aspect by an elliptical incision excising the depression at the base of the thumb. The remaining portion of the proximal phalanx was dead. It was removed, together with the cartilage of the base of the distal phalanx. The bone graft was inserted, its distal end being secured into the reamed-out terminal phalanx, whilst the proximal end was shaped and morticed into the base of the 1st metacarpal using a Hall air drill. A small pin a few millimetres long transfixed the graft and ensured a secure fixation. Plaster immobilisation in a position of function was maintained for 2 months.

Postoperative course was uneventful.

After removing the plaster, function of the thumb progressively recovered. Sensibility in the new pulp is good as regards touch, pin prick and heat and cold. Recognition of small objects is satisfactory.

Three months after the bone graft, the patient was able to resume his normal activities, drive his car and his tractor; he could play tennis and use his thumb for normal everyday functions. The thumb pulp could be actively opposed to the pulp of each finger and his grip was excellent (Figs. 20.5, 20.6, 20.7 and 20.8). The thumb/index

2. *If any attempt to restore the interphalangeal joint is rejected,* the problem becomes much simpler; a flexor tendon graft will be unnecessary and adequate skin cover will enable the insertion of a bone graft between the metacarpal base and the base of the proximal phalanx.

If this plan is adopted:

it is not necessary to reconstruct a long thumb, but rather it is preferable to shorten it, a long rigid thumb being awkward and fragile.

If a tendon graft is not required a suitable gliding surface will not then be necessary to replace skin by a distant flap. Instead, one could use an innervated flap transferred as a one stage procedure from the index finger. Should the skin replacement and bone graft be undertaken at the same time? They should certainly not be combined in this case where there has been sepsis.

Two procedures must therefore be considered, with several months between, so that the second may be performed under

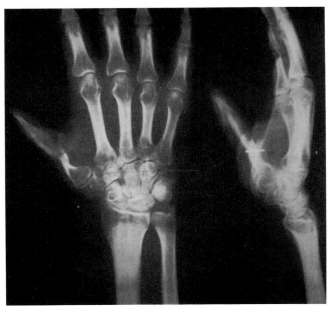

Figure 20.5

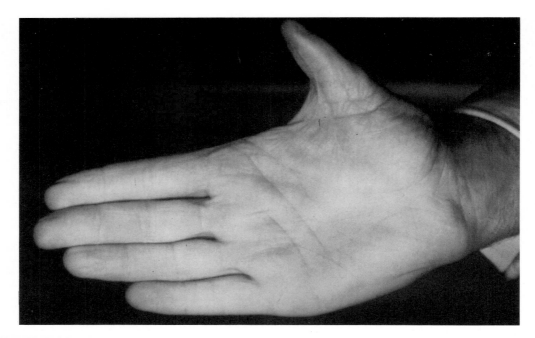

Figure 20.6

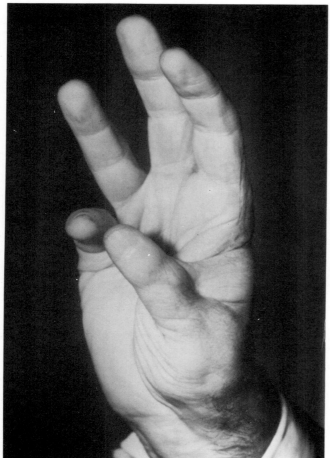

Figure 20.7

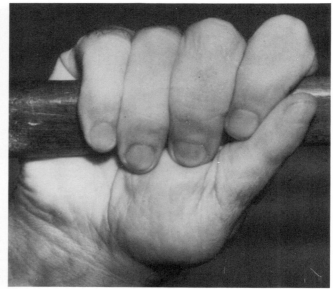

Figure 20.8

web is slightly tethered by the flap transposed from the index finger and should eventually be corrected by a Z-plasty, but the disability is so slight that the patient does not want this to be done.

It seems to us that the interest in this case concerns the discussion as to the choice of treatment and one was able to undertake a relatively modest type of reconstruction by deliberately shortening the thumb and accepting loss of function at the interphalangeal joint. This choice worked out well because the patient regained normal use of the hand after only two operative procedures involving two short periods in hospital.

21. RESULTS AND POSTOPERATIVE MANAGEMENT, RE-EDUCATION AND PSYCHOLOGICAL PROBLEMS IN MUTILATING INJURIES OF THE FINGERS

S. Baux

The ideal treatment of finger injuries, namely a full scale primary repair, is not always feasible except in cases of clear cut linear wounds. Even in these cases, difficulties of bandaging, immobilisation, re-education and rehabilitation do arise in the days and weeks following operation. These difficulties apply even more in multiple injuries, or complicated lacerating or crushing injuries with associated damage to skin, tendon, nerve or bone. It is, therefore, not unusual for the primary operation to be only the first stage of the repair aimed at clean healing, necessitating a further procedure later to complete the reconstruction. The period between these two procedures is of prime importance. The slightest negligence could seriously affect the outcome and inevitably jeopardise the scope of future operative procedures. Too many hand injuries treated initially elsewhere reach specialised hand centres later and although the emergency management has been correct the patients have become apathetic during this secondary period. This apathy is non-surgical in nature, the patient only being remotely connected with hospital, attending for physiotherapy. He may be suffering from psychogenic disturbances and he feels far removed from the slick, brilliant techniques, the elegant flourish and the spectacular success. It is here, however, that the patient's whole future is at stake and depends on small unspectacular measures, on the perseverance of re-education and on his psychological management.

These are the problems with which we would like to deal. In spite of the difficulty presented by their multiple aspects, each lesion and each patient being different, an attempt will be made to classify them showing the results and to establish some principles which may aid treatment.

CLASSIFICATION OF THE IMMEDIATE RESULTS

Following the emergency operation (immediate or delayed for a few hours because of technical reasons), results are either uncomplicated or complicated.

Uncomplicated: with early skin healing.

Problems of re-education and psychological acceptance of the injury or mutilation although easier are nonetheless real and will be examined later.

Complicated: these present difficulties which depend on various pathological features. We may deal with these in turn: necrosis, infection, oedema, stiff joints and other complications.

NECROSIS

There are two types of necrosis: necrosis of digital extremities and necrosis of skin flaps. The first type, whether of arterial or venous origin, may remain dry with resulting mummification of whole or part of a finger, or become infected. Moreover, it is sometimes difficult to judge the extent of the damage and it may be useful to explore each tissue plane before amputating.

Viability of a skin flap is quite a different problem. It has been conceded (J. Gosset, J. Michon) that following emergency skin cover utilising the tissues avulsed by the injury and of doubtful viability, complete survival may occur or there may be complete necrosis or simply epidermal loss with survival of the dermis.

INFECTION

It is generally accepted that infection of the injured hand is rare. It does occur, however, being encouraged by inadequate débridement. Overlooked foreign bodies also predispose to infection. It may accompany sloughing of flaps or wound edges and remain localised; less commonly a deep infection may occur involving synovial sheaths or palmar spaces. Involvement of the bone at the level of amputation is more frequent. The initial cleansing of the wound and the care with which the dressing is applied are more important preventive measures than systemic antibiotics. The latter can do more harm than good and should be condemned. Their use may predispose to subsequent development of resistant infections with formation of adhesions resulting in permanent stiffness.

OEDEMA

Oedema is one of the commonest complications of finger injuries especially those associated with crushing. It affects all the tissues but is naturally predominant on the back of the hand and fingers where the tissue is lax. It spreads to a greater or less extent up the forearm and is accompanied by tension which is painful. This may be because of associated infection but not as a rule. Nevertheless, the results of oedema are serious, leading to disruption of sutures and risk of necrosis due to the internal tourniquet effect which makes the use of appliances or mobilisation difficult. It is a well known fact that it leads to subsequent stiffening of joints probably due to periarticular fibrosis or muscle fibrosis especially of the interosseous muscles where a true localised *Volkmann's* contracture can be seen. A constriction at the site of the dressing or a dependent position for immobilisation will aggravate it. Its prevention should be by an emergency surgical intervention. If stitches are causing tightness they should be removed; sometimes stitches should only be loosely applied or the wound even left open, or for example in the case of the burned hand, a dorsal relaxing incision should be made. Immobilisation in an elevated position with the hand higher than the elbow seemed to us of more value than the repeated use of anti-oedema drugs, in the same way that large wet dressings renewed as required were better than tight ones.

STIFF JOINTS

The risk of stiff joints following the serious complications mentioned may also occur after trivial conditions. Post-operative immobilisation alone, which is necessary, will often produce stiffness.

The inadequacy or even absence of re-education, negligence or half-hearted efforts of the patient are other obvious factors. The part played by psychic factors, which Iselin emphasises, must not be overlooked either, even if one does not go as far as the latter author in this difficult field. We shall return to this subject in discussing methods of re-education. Finally, there is no need to insist on immobilising the hand in a functional position, provided the hand is not allowed to stiffen in a faulty position. All the same, if it is clear as to what position the metacarpophalangeal joints should be placed in, the position for the interphalangeal joints is much more open to discussion, certain persons having even advocated putting them in complete extension. This is an important point since very rapid stiffening of these joints is known to occur.

OTHER TROPHIC DISTURBANCES

Finally, together with these complications, other aspects of trophic disturbances must be emphasised, some limited to the skin (red, sensitive, shiny, smooth), skin appendages (depilation, nails thickened and breaking) and some more generalised, the most marked being the classical stiff, cold, sweating hand with osteoporosis seen in Sudeck's syndrome (atrophy).

PROBLEMS OF TREATMENT

Whether the initial operation was a definitive one with primary reconstruction or only a preparation for a later procedure, the aim of the secondary period, which interests us, is twofold:

To assure skin healing
To prepare for social rehabilitation.

The first heading concerns the management of successive dressings to prepare the hand for further operative procedures at an early stage before the onset of certain complications. The second concerns functional re-education and the psychological reaction of the patient. We shall examine these four points in turn.

SUCCESSIVE DRESSINGS

This is important and often somewhat neglected in descriptions of surgical technique. We intend studying the subject more completely at a later date but for the purpose of this paper it is only possible to enumerate a few principles.

A hand dressing should possess the following qualities:
Be neither heavy nor bulky
Cause no constriction
Provide adequate pressure for haemostasis
Permit movements
Be able to be changed without pain.

The use of tubular stretch material is the most satisfactory means of applying compresses. The latter are best moistened in serum with an added antiseptic. This makes moulding easier. They must not be in direct contact with sutures or raw surfaces.

As far as sutures are concerned, a layer of 'cellophane' can be interposed provided it is never applied circumferentially even by as much as a single filament.

The application of greasy dressings is the only solution for raw surfaces. Whatever the type of wound and contrary to what has long been advocated, it should be inspected. Therefore the dressings must be removed frequently and expeditiously. This is easy since, by taking the precautions we have suggested, it is a painless procedure. One cannot fix precisely the timing of the first dressing or the frequency of changing the dressings. This will depend on clinical examination and questioning the patient, the result of which may necessitate changing the dressing sooner than anticipated. In any case, even in the absence of fever, pain or other disturbing signs, we think it wise to examine the wound every three to four days in case necrosis, with its liability to infection, should develop.

EARLY RE-OPERATION

We do not wish here to open a discussion on the merits of excision, skin cover or secondary amputation. One should recall, however, the value of quickly ridding the patient of a stiff, useless finger whose retention only hinders re-education. It also increases and prolongs the psychological problems.

RE-EDUCATION

The aim of re-education is to restore full function to the hand or at least to prepare it to regain function after repair. The aim must be a supple and painless hand. The means employed vary.

It is usual to think first in terms of active and individual re-education. This may be effected using the Canadian board which most effectively blocks those joints which one is not working on at the time, in order to stimulate mobilisation of other joints. This facilitates individual joint movements. The use of a frame has a similar function and one is also able to encourage movements against resistance by elastic traction or pulley systems. Passive methods, too, must not be neglected since they may be the only ones available, e.g. in the absence of normal motor function when tendons have been divided. They may also be useful to encourage a particular movement. Unfavourable criticism of passive movements is due to their faulty application not to their principle. They cannot replace active methods and they must not produce pain because of the risk of setting up a vicious circle leading to increasing stiffness. Used with circumspection, passive movements prepare the way for active movements. Similarly, massage, is a first class technique which should be adopted in every programme of re-education. Here again, it is a question of gentle, restrained pressure rather than brutal kneading. It enables direct contact with the patient in the true sense. The hand must be warmed and the tissues made supple. The use of emollients such as lanoline and sweet almond oil is also helpful. We have no experience of the mercury bath advocated by some, which has the added advantage of continuous pressure working against resistance which varies according to the depth at which the hand is immersed. It seems to us, however, that this technique cannot altogether replace the initial massage as it lacks human warmth inherent in the act of taking the patient's hand into one's own hands. Working in warm water, however, as soon as healing has occurred is extremely worthwhile and not onerous. Finally, it seems essential to us that this treatment should not be entirely in isolation. Re-education in a group makes use of different games: building things; spillikins; darts; tiddlywinks. This develops a competitive spirit amongst patients and offers a distraction to the mind allowing them to forget their disabilities. This should be an essential feature in re-education and it is a pity that economic factors have sometimes led to their being abondoned (inadequate finances to carry out programmes of group work).

The part played by games seems to us more useful than the occupational therapy often advocated, such as basket-work, at least for men who are bored by it. Needlework, on the contrary, remains an important diversion for women. Re-education in the tasks of every-day life, however, must be systematically pursued. One must at least make use of a system comprising different types of switches, taps, locks, etc. provided they can be installed, as we have seen at Barcelona where there is a real complete apartment set-up. Later, they will graduate to the use of simple tools, e.g. hammer, screwdrivers, pincers. Systematically, therefore, a course of re-education will include a few minutes' massage and warming, individual exercises, group games and limited work-therapy. Personally, we do not use physiotherapy as such. It does not seem to be of any use in the re-education of the hand.

Correcting faulty positions by splintage is, however, of major importance. We agree with Wynn Parry and begin with a succession of static plaster splints, changed as soon as an improvement in position is obtained, before using elastic traction. Recently, instead of plaster, we have been using plastic materials which are easily moulded at reasonable temperatures and being readily re-used their initial somewhat high price can thus be offset.

Together with these methods which, after all, are rather ordinary and conventional, re-education of sensibility must also be stressed. This includes two elements. Firstly, re-education regarding cutaneous contact on a scar, light touch, tapping and percussion as has been used in the treatment of patients with neuromata, are absolutely essential. Secondly, this must be accompanied by the patient seeking out for himself

voluntary contact with various surfaces, initially soft ones, e.g. striking a cushion and then on increasingly hard surfaces. Furthermore, attempts must be made whenever an abnormality exists to re-educate the sense of discrimination using the methods advocated by Wynn Parry. These are based on the recognition of objects with eyes closed. The scope offered by the different techniques used by this author are too often ignored or neglected. We consider that there is another point of major importance namely the collaboration of the surgeon with the therapist. The participation of the latter in consultations, the visiting of the centre by the surgeon, are of first importance and contact between the two should be on a permanent basis. In summing up it is apparent that the programme of re-education overall comes up against certain difficulties: some relate to the state of the injured hand and cannot be eliminated, e.g. need to immobilise fractures, failure of healing. They must be dealt with. Others can be alleviated, e.g. control of pain by analgesics, and the prescribing of tranquillisers for fear and anguish. An essential factor, moreover, is the psychological reaction of the patient with which we shall now deal.

PSYCHOLOGICAL PROBLEMS

The psychological difficulties that can be met amongst patients with hand injuries are two-fold and relate to the patient's previous condition and his reaction to injury.

The patient's previous condition. We shall of course omit from this section the special case of mental patients, since it is uncommon, if not rare, to meet such a situation in routine practice. The psychiatrist's help would then be indispensable. Apart from these cases, three types of patient are often encountered probably because they are more accident prone than the average individual, viz. deprived persons, alcoholics and immigrants.

(a) *By the term 'deprived'* we indicate those people often with apparently normal behaviour pattern but of low I.Q., capable, however, of simple manual work. Their reaction to injury is not easily predicted varying between indifference at one extreme to catastrophic depression at the other. Contact is not always easy to establish but can often develop into complete confidence and trust. It is, moreover, essential to obtain it, for only by this means can their cooperation be counted on and without it, it is impossible to achieve personal initiative or active participation. Particularly open to the influence of those around them, they can change their surgeon, neglect keeping appointments and fail to participate in re-education. The need to guide them in everything may necessitate prolonging their stay in hospital. When discharged they must be given precise instructions and it is essential to make sure that they keep at their work therapy. More important than the surgeon, a remote character to them, are the ancillary staff who can play a dominant part in their management.

(b) *The alcoholic* presents quite a different problem. There is a real risk of delirium tremens in the early days after injury even with simple injuries. We do not intend detailing here its prevention and treatment. Recently, psychological and sociological problems as a result of alcoholism have brought difficulties in re-education. Moreover, the enforced inactivity to which these patients are reduced increases the likelihood of their incidence as more drink is taken to cope with boredom and unemployment. These factors may even induce habit formation in subjects not previously addicted to alcohol. We have had some examples, notably of a young man of 17 who was perfectly normal before his accident. He had a long spell off work as a result of an injury to both his median nerves and he had to undergo treatment for alcoholism. It is important, therefore, to look for intemperate habits or even a tendency towards them in these patients. It may be necessary to simplify treatment, reduce the intervals between operations, get them to take up again some occupation as quickly as possible and keep them occupied before they return to work. The ideal would be to make them undergo treatment for their alcoholism during their convalescence from the injury. This is not impossible but one should not count on it.

(c) *The immigrant* presents another problem, language difficulties tending to make contact difficult. These people, lonely above all, often socially ill-adapted, and having economic problems related to accommodation and food, are particularly vulnerable psychologically speaking. Rejected by their fellow workmates, who often constitute the only community they know, they find themselves completely isolated and up against insoluble problems such as those concerning documents. There is a need here, therefore, to guide them in everything, but it is extremely difficult to gain their confidence. The surgeon and the personnel supervising them remain foreigners and surgical technique is incomprehensible to them. Daily routine is their sole concern and it is often difficult for them to see what the future holds. These problems of social adaptation could take up a whole chapter concerning the association between injury and social conditions. It is not possible to deal with this here except to state that it appears that an individual's reaction to injury is more favourable when he is acquainted with the responsibilities of daily life. Later, we shall see other aspects of this question.

Reactions of the patient to injury. Reactions occur after all injuries, but they are often more marked when concerning the hand, perhaps because of its importance in every-day life and work, perhaps also, because it is the only exposed part of the body constantly seen, it holds a special place in the body make-up. The particularly difficult case of the patient who will not allow his injured hand to be seen would appear to justify this hypothesis. Taking this into account, our experience shows that the results of identical treatment for a particular type of injury varies from one individual to another. Apart from the physical reaction to injury, the patient's psychological reaction also varies, creating an entirely different patient/injury pattern which may appreciably affect the end result. It is difficult to define these different reactions, often of a complex nature in a particular individual and varying from person to person. We will attempt, however, to enumerate the main features which have been encountered with apologies for their necessarily rough and sketchy nature.

1. *Reactions of fear.* These occur first and are most common. They may be present from the start causing difficulty with dressings, remedial applications and re-education. Pain is always present but interpreted differently by individual patients. Fear of pain is often a more powerful restraining influence than the actual pain itself. The outward appearance of the patient is often deceptive as is the understanding that everyone has of himself. The man who thinks he 'can stand pain' is less easy to treat than one who says he 'cannot stand it'. It is of interest that these reactions of fear are generally less marked amongst women but, on the other hand, young people are particularly prey to these reactions. Great care, naturally, must be taken to reduce painful stimuli during dressings, etc. The use of an analgesic provides a useful adjunct, though only relative, because the very fact of using such agents, implants in the patient's mind the need for them and therefore the reality and importance of the pain. This can lead to a certain fixation of natural anxiety.

It would, therefore, appear important to play down this feature.

It should be explained simply to the patient that he must expect to feel a number of disagreeable sensations as an accompaniment to his injury and treatment but not as a central feature. Analgesics should be used only as a temporary measure to tide the patient over the transitory painful period and it should be stressed that this should naturally lead on to a pain-free recovery period. The problem of pain must be approached with much care in the course of the doctor–patient relationship. It should always remain of secondary importance to the main problems which concern return of function and rehabilitation.

2. *Reactions of anxiety and depression.* These are also very common and have many different origins. The psychological trauma of the accident, the phenomena of fear, which we have already mentioned, and anxiety regarding the future, are all involved. Fear of cosmetic disability may be added in some patients, whilst in others it is the finality of the mutilation and the impossibility of imagining anything other than permanent disability. Whatever it may be, the patient only broods about himself whilst continually re-examining himself and his injury. Any active participation in his treatment is out of the question, re-education is impossible the patient protecting his injured hand from all contact. Frequently his general health is also affected by lack of sleep and loss of appetite. Tranquillisers are then absolutely indispensable. They must be prescribed with care, keeping the patient under observation. Physiotherapy might achieve the same result but, generally speaking, recourse to drugs is infinitely simpler and usually efficacious.

3. *Search for personal advantage.* In addition to these involuntary reactions other abnormalities of psychological origin sometimes appear.

Some are concerned simply with the search for ease, the patient settling down comfortably with his disability. A natural tendency to laxness obtrudes leading to an indifference with regard to re-education or improvement. He ceases to participate in re-education if not overtly, at least as soon as supervision ceases. To this attitude there may be added the hope more or less expressed of a 'pension'. The victim of an accident at work is particularly prone to this development, legal aspects encouraging it. Moreover, people often develop it even apart from the fact that self-interest of certain professional men may come into such litigation problems. The opinion of the therapists who know the victim of the accident and the enthusiasm of the injured man in re-education is of prime importance and must influence the surgeon. Treatment is useless. It is a social problem and this can often be solved only be arbitrary decisions about return to work with a permanent pension for partial incapacity. It might then be hoped that the estimate of the patient's economic state thus worked out compared with what he had expected, would alter his outlook and bring about a radical change with a view to his co-operating. Unfortunately, the delays over settling claims are so prolonged that injuries become fixed finally and irreversibly. Certain individuals of a more disinterested nature but of paranoic make-up who are fanatical about justice and compensation, react in exactly the same way.

4. *Infantile regression.* Undoubtedly more common than these features is a superimposed psychological reaction more deeply situated verging on the unconscious but having identical consequences. Many patients find that coping with the responsibilities of daily life, both family and social, requires constant effort. The accident may cause such effort to be suspended and society, in the eyes of the injured man, takes on the role of guardian. Freed from the worry of having to earn a living, able to shelve any problems which, from a practical point of view, he is unable to solve in any case, directed by social workers, taken in hand by doctors and ancillary staff, the individual casts his responsibilities upon them. He finds himself, in some way, reverting to a state of infancy, able to transfer his worries to others and then to free himself from his previous

difficulties. This infantile regression is often present, at least to a certain extent, in patients with hand injuries, in that they can for a time be compulsorily dependent on others for acts of daily life.

The unconscious desire to maintain this state of affairs and not to return to the arena of responsibilities hinders, or can even cut across, rehabilitation. These cases are obviously difficult or even impossible to treat under the present set-up. They can be solved only by compromises tacitly accepted on both sides with only moderate success. The participation of a qualified psychiatrist used to dealing with this type of problem would alone enable progress to be made. At present, the collaboration of an intelligent therapist can be of help, however, when he agrees to accept, in addition to his duties, the 'role of mother', making use of this regression to rehabilitate the patient and gradually restore him to a state when he can again resume his own responsibilities.

CONCLUSION

To sum up, all these psychological problems pose more questions than they solve. If the use of tranquillisers is a recent and beneficial acquisition, the other possible therapeutic measures are little employed doubtless due to lack of time and preparation. However this may be, it seemed of importance to us to try to sort out the different questions posed by the postoperative complications following the initial management of the injured hand. We do not claim to have propounded all the problems, still less to have found miraculous solutions to them, but it seems of prime importance to take an interest in them, to seek closer collaboration between all those concerned in their treatment and to establish a really sound doctor–patient relationship.

I

22. TREATMENT OF PAINFUL AMPUTATION STUMPS

F. Iselin

Is it possible to prevent painful amputation stumps?

Indeed, the carrying out of a technically perfect amputation can eliminate the problem of painful sequelae but this is not always true and the best amputations can become unbearably painful.

It is necessary indeed to distinguish clearly two groups of very different cases in both their origin and results.

(1) The stumps may be painful because of obvious lesions or (2) they may be painful without any apparent reason.

In 34 cases operated on between 1965 and 1969 there were 17 in the first category and 17 in the second. Treatment of the 17 stumps in which there were lesions present has produced the following results: 13 cures, 3 improvements, 1 failure. For the 17 purely painful stumps: 6 cures, 4 improvements, 7 failures.

In the former group, the way in which the stump is re-fashioned is the essential thing, the way the nerve is dealt with being less important. In the 17 cases we have undertaken:

3 further resections with recovery

4 diathermy treatment with 3 cures and one improvement

3 bone implantations by the *Teneff* technique with one cure, one improvement and one failure

7 no treatment with 7 recoveries.

The series of purely painful stumps set problems which will require much more consideration. It is a known fact the *Nanterre* School's views are somewhat unorthodox concerning the aetiology of painful stumps. We think that a subjective factor alone, largely inherent in the personality of the patient, is able to explain the onset and development of this truly painful condition. With this concept in mind, let us recall certain facts:

The infrequency of these painful stumps. All statistics give a lower figure than 6 per cent. None of 70 amputated fingers at *Nanterre* in the last 5 years has developed a painful stump.

Their absence in children. All our cases operated on were in adults, the youngest being 17.

The wide range of times at which a painful stump develops after amputation. In our 17 cases, 5 said they had pain the day after amputation and of the others the delay varied between 6 and 14 months.

The absence of a constant association between the existence of a neuroma and of pain. In our 17 cases, we have only demonstrated one or more neuromata in 12 of them and in one of these where there were two painful stumps a neuroma was present in the one but not the other.

In studying these cases one can distinguish two groups of differing severity:

Those with genuine pain : simply painful stumps, particularly when knocked, and only to a limited extent occurring spontaneously, with frequent sensations like electric shocks and phantom limb sensation which may or may not be painful. Eleven out of the 17 came into this category.

They have a better prognosis—6 cures, 4 improvements and 1 failure.

The painful syndrome : less common, characterised by constant pain, true causalgia producing trophic changes in finger and hand and also causing changes such as redness or blueness, oedema and excessive sweating in the finger. There is a constant association with psychological disturbances. The disastrous prognosis is indicated by our results—six cases, six failures.

Treatment varies, therefore, according to the type of painful stump:

For those with genuine pain. Surgical treatment was beneficial in 10 out of 11 cases of which 6 were cures.

The following methods were used:

Bone implantation as described by *Teneff* in 7 cases with 2 cures, 4 improvements and 1 failure.

There was one further recovery after a cosmetic amputation.

We agree with Razemon that cosmetic amputation is a good method of treating these painful stumps.

Bipolar electro-coagulation as described by J. Gosset has been used in 4 cases with 3 cures and one improvement. This latter technique has now, in fact, become our routine procedure.

We always put the patient on tranquillisers when undergoing this treatment to avoid the development of a pain fixation and also the possibility of a case with genuine pain developing into the so-called painful syndrome.

For the painful syndrome : the frequency of failures indicates that they should not be treated surgically. We first tried the effect of tranquillisers and minor procedures such as percussion or hammering under local anaesthesia which enabled the patient to dissociate his painful finger from his psychogenic control.

The failures were referred to a neuro-psychiatrist. We think that all attempts at further local treatment are not only doomed to failure but may even make the condition worse. We have already mentioned this twice and we feel that these procedures aggravate the psychological aspect of the condition. It would appear that these patients have nothing to gain from neurosurgery.

These quasi-desperate cases are fortunately rare and preventative measures might be useful, for example, psychological management of the patient from the time of his original amputation.

The least one can do, as we have done, is to give the patients tranquillisers routinely in all cases.

CONCLUSION

In a series of 34 painful amputation stumps seen over a period of 4 years, corrective surgery has led to recovery or improvement as follows: 16 out of 17 cases where the stumps were faulty; 10 out of 17 purely painful stumps. It is significant that the 10 cures or improvements were seen in the 11 stumps classified in the genuine pain group whereas in the other group ('painful syndrome') out of 6 cases there were 6 failures and 2 of these were made even worse.

It is important, therefore, to recognise this latter group of cases in which operative treatment, in our opinion, is absolutely contra-indicated.

23. COSMETIC PROBLEMS IN THE RECONSTRUCTION OF FINGER-STUMPS

C. Dufourmentel

Cosmetic problems concerning the hands, especially those related to amputations of the fingers, are important. Admittedly, function in a hand is more important than its cosmetic appearance, but with certain people, this latter feature does count considerably. This applies particularly to girls and young women. Men, however, specially those of the professional class, are not exempt. It is not uncommon for patients with perfect function to avoid using an unsightly finger and hide it to prevent those around them from seeing it. An example of this occurred in one of my patients who had been operated on for radiodermatitis: this was a dentist on whom I had to excise the skin from the dorsum of all four fingers of his left hand. The nail of the index finger together with its matrix had to be removed, but ugly nail remnants regrew: function in the finger was perfectly normal. This practitioner, however, preferred not to use the finger which he kept flexed in his palm, holding his instruments only with his thumb and middle finger so that his patients would not see his index finger.

There are instances, therefore, where the restoration of a mutilated finger, as aesthetically as possible, is imperative. One must beware, however, of certain patients who are psychologically unsuited to reconstruction. They will demand the impossible, will never be satisfied, and will always bear a grievance against a surgeon who is not able to fulfil their expectations. However, provided cases are carefully selected with clear indications and assuming the patients understand the possibilities and their limitations, satisfactory results both from the surgeon's and patients' point of view, may be obtained.

In our opinion, there are three types of case in which the indications for treatment are quite different. These are:
1. Total amputation of a finger
2. Partial amputation of a finger, preserving a sufficiently useful stump, but without preserving the nail
3. Amputation through the nail.

1. TOTAL AMPUTATION OF A FINGER

The aim in this case must be a hand with three contiguous fingers and the thumb but leaving no gap between adjacent fingers. In general, such a hand is very pleasing to the eye, and it may not be immediately obvious at a glance, that a finger is missing. Provision of such a three-fingered hand is easy when amputating the index or little finger. It is only necessary to complete the finger amputation by removal of the corresponding metacarpal but, preferably, leaving its base cut obliquely. This will leave a smooth line tailing off from metacarpal to carpus.

The problem is more difficult with the middle and ring finger.

Generally speaking, with the ring finger, amputation of the head and distal part of the metacarpal is adequate. The adjacent little and middle fingers can be approximated. Admittedly, this does result in a slight rotation of the metacarpal axes causing a somewhat exaggerated convergence of the two fingers when they are flexed. However, this is never awkward or unsightly. On the other hand, resection of the 3rd metacarpal is followed by a more marked rotation of the 2nd and 4th rays which is distinctly awkward and results in overlapping of the index and ring fingers on flexion. In this case, therefore, let us transfer the index to take the place of the middle finger. Although this is a more major procedure, it is justified by the functional and cosmetic results.

2. PARTIAL AMPUTATION OF A FINGER WITH LOSS OF THE NAIL

These cases include amputations through the proximal and middle phalanges, through the interphalangeal joints and certain amputations of the most proximal part of the distal phalanx. In these cases, the best results appear to me to be achieved by prostheses. *Pillet* has produced excellent prostheses which give a very satisfactory appearance. These prostheses, made of plastic material, end proximally in a kind of glove finger which fits over the stump. The junction of normal skin with the prosthesis is readily masked by the wearing of a ring. Needless to say, such a device is more easily used in the case of amputation of the ring or little finger. This technique sometimes necessitates surgical revision of a stump which is too bulky. The appearance would be ugly if the prosthesis had to fit onto a large stump whose diameter it would increase still further. It is, therefore, quite legitimate to reduce the soft tissue or even the bone in these cases. Certain patients are unwilling to accept a prosthesis and prefer amputation of the whole digital ray closing the space between the fingers. This has been discussed under the previous heading.

3. AMPUTATIONS THROUGH THE NAIL

The following instances occur. Firstly, in the more distal amputations of the finger and nail, the nail is worth preserving. Secondly, amputation occurs through the matrix so that a nail remains but is of very poor quality. Finally, amputation has been accompanied by crushing of the matrix so that growth of the nail is too poor for it to be of any use. In the first case, the nail can be preserved and there are several operations which may be undertaken depending on the type of the deformity. The simplest deformity is that which consists of a wide, short nail. In this case, all that is required is resection of two lateral strips of this wide nail together with the corresponding part of the matrix and, of course, the nail bed. The advancement of the skin of the nail setting to the inner edge of the resection, produces a very narrow nail whose length/width ratio approaches normal. Certainly, the finger is a little shortened, but the cosmetic result is usually acceptable.

The problem is much more difficult when the injured finger presents three associated deformities. Firstly, there is widening and shortening of the nail. Secondly, there is the parrot's beak deformity of the nail, where the nail instead of lying in its normal position comes to lie more or less horizontally over the finger end. Finally, the whole finger end is wide in relation to its length. The widening may be due solely to soft tissue or to bony overgrowth at the divided end of the phalanx (Fig. 23.1).

The three elements of this deformity can be corrected by an operation which we originally described (Dufourmentel, 1963) and which is undertaken as follows. The excessive width of the nail is reduced by a resection of nail, matrix and nail bed on either side. The parrot's beak deformity of the nail and its excessive shortness can be corrected by taking back the nail and its matrix and bed all in one piece. To do this, we extend the two lateral excisions by two longitudinal incisions for at least a centimetre and a half beyond the root of the nail (Fig. 23.2). On the deep aspect of the nail bed and the flap raised by these two incisions, we dissect deeply to the level of the bone to ensure a good blood supply to the skin and nail flap raised (Fig. 23.3). By folding the proximal part of this flap, it will be possible to shift the nail back and apply it to the end of the phalanx (Fig. 23.4). Naturally, this will produce a swelling at the level of the base of the flap, but this swelling usually subsides spontaneously. If not, it may be reduced at a subsequent operation. Having shifted the nail back, a defect is left distally which must be covered. For this we use two lateral flaps raised on either side of the proximally based median flap (Figs 23.2 and 23.3). The lateral flaps are then transposed at right angles and sutured to each other, covering the whole anterior part of the dorsal aspect of the finger (Fig. 23.4). They thus provide for closure of the skin defect resulting from shifting the nail back and, at the same time, give additional support for the latter and slight lengthening of the finger end. Finally, the defects created on both sides of the nail by the nail bed reduction and the raising of the two lateral flaps which are transposed, reduce the bulk of the finger end. This is a good way, in fact, of resecting subcutaneous tissue or even reducing bony prominences at the end of the phalanx. Skin closure at the end of the operation moulds the finger tip making it more shapely. The appearance has been markedly improved as a result of this operation (Fig. 23.5). Admittedly, it is not possible to

restore the part to normal, but the results have certainly been encouraging.

The problem becomes more difficult when the amputation passes through the most proximal part of the nail, either the nail fold or even entirely in the matrix. A nail of sorts remains, maybe only fragments, but the quality is poor and cannot be used for refashioning a normal nail. In this case we use a procedure derived from those described by Buncke and Gonzales (1962) and by McCash (1963) the aim of which is to prepare a suitable bed for attaching an artificial nail. By this method we have had some satisfactory results but also some failures. We feel there is scope here to perfect a technique. The principle consists of resecting the whole of what remains of nail and matrix to prevent any further growth of unsightly nail remnants. The finger-tip must also be modelled to a slender form comparable to the normal. Finally, a nail-bed and setting is constructed to which an artificial nail can be applied. To make this nail-bed and setting, the skin from the dorsal aspect of the finger is removed over an area to correspond with that required for the new nail. The edges of the excised area are undermined to create a kind of pocket into which the artificial nail will eventually be fitted. A thin skin graft 0·3 millimetre in thickness is then applied to the nail-bed and setting including the pocket which is lined by turning the graft back on itself. In order to maintain the graft-lined pocket, an artificial nail is introduced or a thick sheet of silastic covered in a layer of dressing.

It is essential, on the one hand, to obtain a good take of this graft and on the other to maintain a good, deep pocket by means of a prosthesis over a long period, otherwise it will gradually be transformed into a simple gutter and eventually disappear altogether.

Our failures have been due, either to unsatisfactory take of the graft, to infection which prevented maintaining the prosthesis in place, negligence of the patient or, finally, to a bad fit of the prosthesis. However, in four cases, we obtained a good pocket into which the artificial nail fitted accurately. We had hoped that this pocket would spontaneously hold a prosthesis which we had made slightly thicker in its proximal part so that it might be firmly wedged in and remain stable. In fact, this did not work out and we have always had to use gum to fix the artificial nail in its new bed. Satisfactory adhesive agents now exist but they are not tolerated by all patients and it is advisable for the prosthesis to be worn only part of the time, not constantly.

This operation might equally well be used in cases where there is no true shortening of the finger, simply mutilation of its tip destroying the nail or damaging it so seriously that it is not worth preserving. Possible techniques for reconstruction here have not yet been perfected, but we feel it is worth mentioning them as they appear to offer considerable promise.

The ideal is, undoubtedly, to attempt the reconstruction of the damaged finger-tip at the time of the primary amputation. A recent article by Beasley (1969) described a very ingenious technique for avoiding the parrot's beak deformity in amputations through the nail. It involves using a thenar flap, raised in the conventional way, to repair the amputated finger tip in

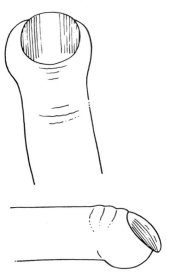

Figure 23.1
Injured finger tip with amputation through the nail: widening of finger tip; widening of the nail; shortening of both these structures; parrot's beak deformity of the nail.

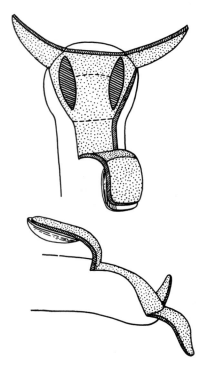

Figure 23.3
The three flaps have been raised. The shaded ellipses represent the soft tissues and bony fragments which must be removed to reduce the bulk of the finger-tip.

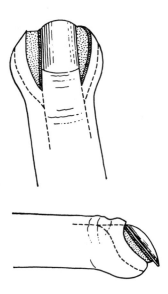

Figure 23.2
First step of operation: reducing the width of the nail. The dotted line outlines the three flaps: the median which includes the nail, nail bed and matrix, and the lateral which are purely skin flaps based distally.

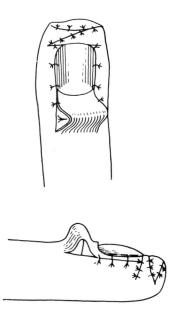

Figure 23.4
Folding back the median flap at its base allows setting back of the nail. The transposition of the lateral flaps in front of the nail closes the resulting defect. They maintain growth of the nail and prevent the parrot's beak deformity. Closing the lateral defects maintains the reshaped finger-tip.

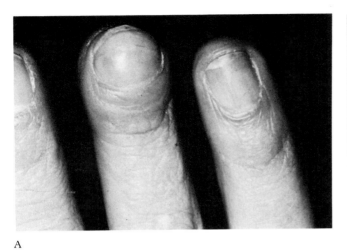

A

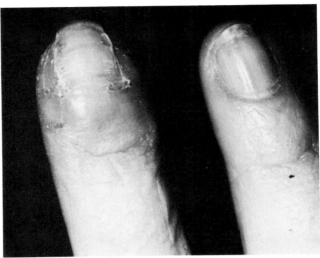

B

Figure 23.5
A, Typical injury to tip of left middle finger. Compare the nail with that of the adjacent index finger.
B, Six weeks after operation. Note the already considerable reduction in postoperative swelling at the base of the median flap.

a sausage-shaped manner. The special feature of this flap is, however, that the end of the flap is left projecting beyond the finger-tip and is not sutured to cover the dorsal defect on the finger. Two to three weeks later, when the flap has taken, the author divides the base of the flap, and sets it in to the palmar aspect after removal of excess subcutaneous tissue giving a smooth roundness to the finger pulp. On the dorsal aspect, he does not attempt to inset the flap to cover the loss of substance. The acute angle at the dorsal surface of the finger-tip is created by severing the redundant tip of the flap in the plane of the nail-bed and using the skin of the amputated distal flap as a full-thickness graft to close the dorsal wound. This may be replaced later by a nail-bed graft from the big toe and to which the growing nail adheres. The support for the nail also prevents the parrot's beak deformity and, by remodelling the nail-bed, widening of the nail is also prevented. The author claims that it is unnecessary to bone-graft the finger-tip, the thenar flap itself providing sufficient support for the growing nail.

We have never tried this technique. We propose employing it in spite of a certain reluctance on our part to use a palmar flap.

SUMMARY

Although perhaps appearing a minor problem, the masking of cosmetic defects resulting from finger amputations seems to us worthwhile.

Total amputation of a finger will be hardly noticeable if the mutilated hand can be transformed into a hand with three contiguous fingers and a thumb.

Partial amputations, leaving a sufficient length of stump, but where there is no possibility of nail reconstruction, are best disguised by a prosthesis in the form of a glove finger.

Amputations through the nail are treated by reconstructive measures aimed at reducing the width of the nail and finger-tip, and setting back the nail. If this last procedure is not feasible, an artificial nail, fixed on a skin graft and in a reconstructed nail setting, will give a very reasonable result.

BIBLIOGRAPHY

BEASLEY, R. W. (1969). Reconstruction of amputated finger tip. *Plastic and Reconstructive Surgery*, **44,** 349.
BUNCKE, H. J. Jr. & GONZALES, R. J. (1962). Fingernail Reconstruction. *Plastic and Reconstructive Surgery*, **30,** 452.
DUFOURMENTEL, C. (1963). Correction chirurgicale des extrémités digitales en massue. *Anm. Chir., plast.*, **44,** 349.
MCCASH, C. R. (1963). Treatment of fingernail deformities. *Proceedings of IIIrd International Congress of Plastic Surgery*. Washington. Amsterdam: Excerpta Medica.
PEACOCK, E. E. (1962). Metacarpal transfer following amputation of a central digit. *Plastic and Reconstructive Surgery*, **29,** 345.

24. THE KRUKENBERG OPERATION

R. Tubiana

The aim of this operation is to fashion the forearm into an active pincer, the arms of which are covered with sensitive soft tissue.

This operation was devised by Krukenberg in 1917. It was mainly used in Germany during the First World War. Kallio in Finland (1948) described the technique and analysed his results. In spite of its spectacular nature, this ingenious procedure lapsed into oblivion and has been employed in only a few centres, e.g. Germany (Simon, 1961), Italy (Zanoli, 1957) and the United States (Swanson, 1964).

At the Orthopaedic Clinic of l'Hôpital Cochin, Paris, R. Merle D'Aubigné, P. Maurer and I have carried out this excellent procedure on several occasions.

TECHNIQUE

The operation is performed under tourniquet.

1. INCISIONS

We use two skin flaps.

(a) The *anterior* incision is begun three finger-breadths below the elbow medial to the long axis and extends radially and distally one centimetre from the radial border of the forearm to the extremity of the stump forming a wide flap based on the ulnar side.

(b) *Posteriorly* the incision is the reverse, forming a flap based radially. An alternative is to use an approach similar to that employed by Bunnell in the treatment of syndactyly, with one or two V-flaps based proximally to form the commissure.

The skin flaps are raised with the underlying deep fascia.

2. MUSCLE DISSECTION

(a) *Anteriorly:* the first step is to expose pronator teres which marks the upper limit of separation of the two arms of the pincer.

One dissects between pronator teres and palmaris longus and then splits flexor superficialis between the bellies going to the middle and ring fingers. The muscular arcade is divided.

On a deeper plane one then goes between flexor profundus on the ulnar side and flexor pollicis longus radially.

(b) *Posteriorly:* the common extensor is split between its heads of origin. One then passes between extensor digiti minimi on the ulnar side and extensor indicis proprius, the thumb extensors and abductor pollicis longus on the radial side.

Both surfaces of the interosseous membrane are then exposed.

3. RESECTION OF NERVES

The median nerve is divided as it emerges from pronator teres and the distal end is resected well clear of the skin suture line. The posterior interosseous nerve is preserved.

The interosseous vessels are ligated at the proximal part of the interosseous membrane and resected.

The motor nerves are divided away from the ends of the pincer but the radial and ulnar arteries are ligated as far distally as possible.

4. DIVISION OF THE INTEROSSEOUS MEMBRANE AND SEPARATION OF THE BONES

The interosseous membrane is removed completely. The bones may now be separated widely, by 10 to 12 cm in the adult when they are cut just proximal to the upper border of pronator quadratus.

The optimal length of the arms of the pincer is 12 to 15 cm (Fig. 24.1). If longer the blood supply to their extremities may be inadequate. (This length does not include the distance between the commissure of the pincer and the fold of the elbow.)

Sometimes one may have to accept much shorter arms; we have at times fashioned very short Krukenberg pincers measuring only 7 cm which nevertheless have been agile and

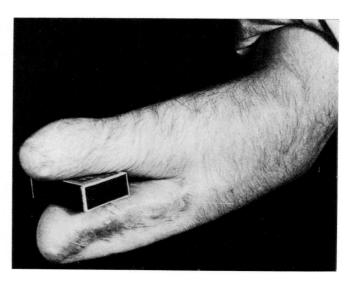

Figure 24.1
Result of Krukenberg operation showing optimal length of pincer.

126

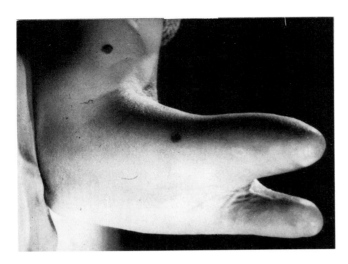

Figure 24.2
Short pincer following Krukenberg reconstruction which, nevertheless, has useful function.

sensitive (Fig. 24.2). The muscles activating the pincers are mostly proximal. It is the radius which moves in relation to the ulna. To open the pincer it is necessary to use the abductors of the radius, i.e. biceps and brachioradialis, the radial group, and to close the pincer, the adductors of the radius, i.e. pronator teres and supinator. To achieve a strong pincer movement it is essential to stabilise the ulna by use of triceps, brachialis and anconeus.

The other forearm muscles have only an accessory function, therefore one should not hesitate to excise them if they are too bulky to allow easy skin closure. One may discard first the muscles acting on the thumb which are the least useful.

Tendons which have been kept are divided into the two groups and are sutured to the extremities of the bones.

5. CLOSURE OF THE SOFT TISSUES

The tourniquet is released, haemostasis achieved and the skin flaps are wrapped around the two arms of the pincer. It is imperative that the skin covering opposing surfaces of the pincer has sensation. The soft tissues should be sutured to periosteum to give stability to the grip.

The commissure of the pincer may be closed using a V-flap as in the repair of syndactyly.

When two large skin flaps based anteriorly and posteriorly have been fashioned, the anterior one is introduced between the two bones over the pronator teres and its outer upper angle is sutured to the corresponding angle of the posterior defect. The inner upper angle of the posterior flap is likewise sutured to the corresponding angle of the anterior defect. Any residual deficiencies are made good by the use of free skin grafts.

6. REHABILITATION

This is begun immediately after the skin has healed soundly, during the second week. Every effort must be made to mobilise

the radius whilst holding the ulnar arm still, stabilised by the antagonistic action of triceps and brachialis. Opening the pincer should not be done by a supinating movement, nor its closure by a pronating movement, as these interfere with precision of the grip. The physiotherapist should initially maintain the ulna immobile, the elbow in slight flexion, and encourage the patient to move the radius in a sagittal plane in neutral pronation-supination (Maurer, 1976).

RESULTS

Functional results are on the whole very satisfactory. The patients use their pincers for all every-day functions.

They are able to take small objects from their pockets which are identified by touch and to hold larger objects measuring up to 10 cm in diameter. If power at the extremity of the pincer does not exceed 2 to 3 kg, it is greatly in excess of this at its base; with the elbow flexed it may be 8 to 10 kg. Sensation at the extremity of the pincer improves gradually and Swanson (1964) has observed, in the child, tactile discrimination comparable with that of a normal hand. Two-point discrimination (*Weber's test*) may be as little as 4 mm although this may be as much as 1 cm in normal forearm skin.

The unsightly appearance of the pincer remains a problem, less so for the patient, usually delighted with the functional result of his operation, than for those around him. The appearance may be disguised when socially necessary by a hand prosthesis which can be activated by the arms of the Krukenberg pincer.

INDICATIONS

The Krukenberg operation is indicated in cases of congenital or traumatic amputation of the hand.

In congenital amputations, Swanson (1964) advises early operation, from the age of 2 years, with retention of a digit where one exists at the extremity of one arm of the pincer, as this may improve precision movements. He has obtained excellent results.

In traumatic amputations, the Krukenberg operation gives good results if the soft tissues are not damaged: in particular if the nerve supply of the skin covering the extremities of the pincer is not impaired. It is therefore an operation which is rarely possible following burns. It is also essential that the tissues should be supple, well-vascularised and the muscles in good condition.

One must be cautious when advising this operation following amputation after an electric burn or ischaemia.

In unilateral amputations where the remaining hand ensures the patient's independence, a prosthesis is usually preferred to an operation which is only designed to provide extra help. On the other hand, when the patient is young and has an occupation which demands sensibility of both his upper extremities, it is the Krukenberg pincer which offers the maximum scope for function. If one hand has been amputated and where the remaining hand is seriously handicapped, the Krukenberg operation on the amputated limb is plainly indicated to achieve a wide grasp and strong grip.

In cases where both hands have been amputated the Krukenberg operation seems the best approach, performed either bilaterally, or unilaterally in association with a prosthesis on the other side. This must be discussed with the patient and showing him a film of an operated case is most valuable. Bilateral amputees treated by this technique regain total independence. They are able to wash themselves, dress themselves, cook, feed themselves, drive a car, write, sew, or type using a small pusher adapted to one of the arms of the pincer. The fashioning of a sensitive pincer is particularly necessary in blind patients. It is in those cases, which unfortunately are not exceptional, where both hands and eyes have been damaged by explosives that the Krukenberg operation is particularly indicated.

BIBLIOGRAPHY

KALLIO, K. E. (1948). Recent advance in Krukenberg's operation. *Acta chirurgica scandinavica*, **97**, 165–188.

KRUKENBERG, H. (1917). *Uber Plastische Umwertung von Amputationstumpfen*. Stuttgart: Ferdinand Enke.

MAURER, P. (1976). Personal communication.

SIMON, P. (1961). Modalitaten des wieder eingetretenen Hautgefuhls an Bauchhaut-Plastiken von Krukenberg-Greifarmen. *Monatsschrift für Unfallheilkunde und Versicherurgsmedizin*, **64**, 429–433, H. 11. Springer-Verlag.

SWANSON, A. B. (1964). The Krukenberg procedure in the juvenile amputee. *Journal of Bone and Joint Surgery*, **46-A,** 1540–1549.

TUBIANA, R. (1969). Repair of bilateral hand mutilations. *Plastic and Reconstructive Surgery*, **44,** 323–330.

ZANOLI, R. (1957). Krukenberg-Putti Amputation-Plasty. *Journal of Bone and Joint Surgery*, **39-B,** 230–232.

25. *FUNCTIONAL PROSTHESES FOR THE MUTILATED HAND*

J. Xenard and J-M. Paquin

After a major hand mutilation, the following possibilities are open to the patient:

Use of a functional prosthesis,

Use of a dress hand for social purposes,

Use of his bare stump.

The choice of prosthesis will depend on the patient's personal requirements and on the type of job he has to do. The role of therapists, surgeons and specialists in physical medicine at this stage will be to provide information to assist the patients.

USE OF THE BARE STUMP

The mutilated hand is kept covered with a woollen cap or a dressing, or simply kept in the pocket. For most of the time, the stump is not used and the patient develops dexterity in the other hand which enables him to achieve satisfactory independence. He will then use fittings for certain complicated manoeuvres requiring both hands.

However, there will be many manual jobs requiring two hands which he will be unable to manage.

Sometimes the stump is used for securing things for pinching or holding.

DRESS HANDS FOR SOCIAL PURPOSES

In certain cases these can be of real functional value. Pillet's work on these prostheses is well known.

TRUE FUNCTIONAL PROSTHESES

In major hand mutilations, one should mention the subject of prostheses at an early stage. These prostheses which have often been of a repellent aspect, should be designed to enable that type of prehension which will be most frequently used in the patient's job. There are different groups of functional prostheses depending on the nature of the injury (Fig. 25.1).

REMAINING INTACT THUMB

If the remaining thumb lacks sensation, it is useless however mobile it may be because it is unable to ensure support against the prosthetic appliance. It is preferable to sacrifice it at this stage.

If the thumb, whilst possessing sensation, is stiff and immobile, it is again useless and must either be mobilised or amputated.

When the hand possesses only a thumb, it will be used if the latter has sensation and mobility and also if there is an

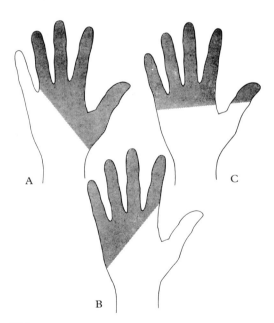

Figure 25.1
A, Radial hemiamputation.
B, Surviving thumb—ulnar amputation.
C, Transverse amputation.

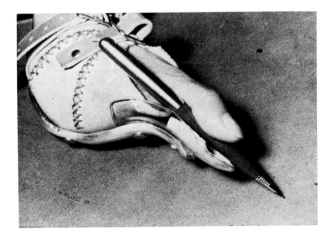

Figure 25.2
Appliance for loss of ulnar part of hand with surviving thumb.

129

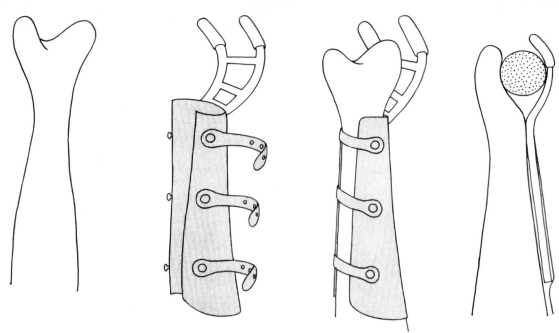

Figure 25.3
Appliance for transverse amputation of the hand.

adequate second metacarpal remnant against which the grip can be made effective. In the absence of this, the thumb is used as a hook.

The prosthesis is composed of a socket and a terminal fitting. Initially, a study socket is made in plastic. One fits the necessary terminal appliance and observes its use in the occupational therapy department and the clinic.

The skin must be in perfect condition so that the stump may support the prosthesis. There must be no residual hypersensitivity.

As a result of observations made in the clinic, adjustments are made to the socket and a more permanent appliance is made in synthetic material, leather, steel or aluminium (Fig. 25.2).

These appliances restore prehension by opposition to the pulp just proximal to the tip, i.e. the thumb pulp appliance (pinch grip).

The lateral pinch is made between the pulp of the thumb and the radial edge of the prosthesis.

Grasp will be in the nature of a hook, the thumb closing the hook.

TRANSVERSE AMPUTATION OF THE HAND

However long the stump may be, it will be of little use because only bimanual prehension and direct support are left.

1. If the stump is very short, the appliance is the same as for amputations of the distal forearm. The socket is modified to allow for wrist movements and, also, pronation and supination. A pincer or hand is fixed to the socket. Active opening of this is achieved by forward movement of the shoulder transmitted by a harness. Closure is passive, the strength of which can be controlled.

2. If the stump is longer, one then fits an appliance made up of a sheath or cuff (in plastic or leather) allowing for free movement of the wrist (Fig. 25.3) and by fitting the branching form of which allows general or more specific use. Sometimes, one may be asked to make attachments for milking cows, for using woodwork tools and other specialised jobs.

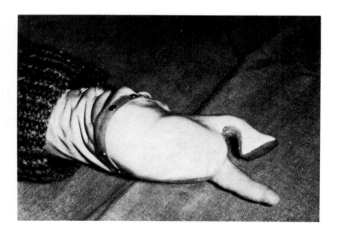

Figure 25.4
Appliance of radial hemiamputation. Pinch grip completed by the little finger.

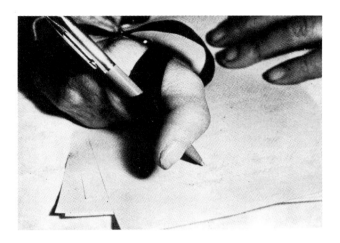

Figure 25.5
Appliance modified for appropriate function.

One may make use of wrist flexion to obtain prehension between the stump and a fixed attachment on the forearm.

These appliances can have different fittings adapted for the same socket, or even for knives, forks, pens.

AMPUTATION OF RADIAL PART OF THE HAND

The little finger remains with part of the ring. If the little finger is mobile or possesses sensation, it may be of considerable value. If this is not the case it is better removed. The mobile little finger provides a hook, which though rather weak is nevertheless useful.

If the dominant hand is not involved the majority of such partial amputees manage to use the dominant hand adequately without the use of a prosthesis on the other hand.

If the dominant hand is involved an opposition appliance is made and in addition is modified with a minimal socket. This double hook or specialised pinch appliance enables a grip in conjunction with the little finger (Fig. 25.4). There must be a freedom for design with such an appliance. Its specific requirements in each case must be studied in action at a specialised centre and then appropriately modified to suit each case (Fig. 25.5).

The appearance of such an appliance is extremely unsightly and it will only be used by a patient if it significantly improves his function, whether at his job or in every-day life.

Only one-third of the patients fitted with such an appliance continue to use it and these attend regularly for repairs or renewal.

The fittings most frequently used are those necessary for driving a car.

INDEX